USING THE BODIES OF THE DEAD

Using the Bodies of the Dead

Legal, ethical and organisational dimensions of organ transplantation

NORA MACHADO
University of Uppsala, Sweden

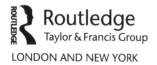

Routledge
Taylor & Francis Group

LONDON AND NEW YORK

First published 1998 by Dartmouth and Ashgate Publishing

Reissued 2018 by Routledge
2 Park Square, Milton Park, Abingdon, Oxon, OX14 4RN
52 Vanderbilt Avenue, New York, NY 10017

Routledge is an imprint of the Taylor & Francis Group, an informa business

Publisher's Note
The publisher has gone to great lengths to ensure the quality of this reprint but points out that some imperfections in the original copies may be apparent.

Disclaimer
The publisher has made every effort to trace copyright holders and welcomes correspondence from those they have been unable to contact.

A Library of Congress record exists under LC control number:

ISBN 13: 978-1-138-38704-1 (hbk)
ISBN 13: 978-0-429-42645-2 (ebk)

Contents

List of Figures

List of Tables

Preface

This work, building on earlier studies of Renée Fox, Bernward Joerges, Roberta Simmons, among others, explores in depth the multi-dimensional and highly elusive character of organ transplantation as a social, technical, and cultural phenomenon. I have tried to bridge theoretically and methodologically the thick cultural analyses of Fox and Simmons, on the one hand, and the socio-technical perspective of Joerges, on the other. I introduce and apply a range of new concepts and models in analysing organ transplantation systems: the dissonances that appear to be endemic to these systems; the particular function of a number of hospital roles, rituals, and discourses in dealing with such dissonance and related conflict; the legal and normative regulation of body part extraction and allocation in large-scale systems; the cognitive and moral dilemmas which physicians, nurses, and next-of-kin face in the use of the bodies of the dead.

In examining the ethical aspects of organ transplantation, I try to avoid the highly decontextualized treatment of bio-medical ethics that characterise a great deal of the philosophical approach.

Much of my theoretical work is of a general character and should be of considerable interest even to those not engaged in issues of organ transplantation or bio-medical developments.

Nora Ines Machado

Florence, Italy
March 31, 1998

Acknowledgements

I am grateful to Beth Maina Ahlberg, Tom R. Burns, Björn Eriksson and Renée Fox for careful reading and critical suggestions of earlier versions of substantial parts of this manuscript. I also want to thank my colleagues from the Uppsala Theory Circle Seminars and others who have read parts of this work and provided constructive criticisms and advice: Bo Andersson, Torbjörn Bilgård, Håkan Johansson, Göran Lanz, John Lilja, Mohammadrafi Mahmoodian, Anders Olsson, Pablo Suarez, Per Sundberg, Thorlief Petterson, and Hans Zetterberg.

I am also indebted to Dr. Lars Frödin and to Christina Bergström at the Transplantation Centre of Uppsala Academic Hospital for their openness and support; and also to interviewees and hospital personnel in a number of Swedish units who gave me their time and attention. Also, many thanks to Eurotransplant and Scandiatransplant, in particular to Frank Pedersen at Scandiatransplant, for being so service-minded, even for someone like myself who was not a client.

Finally, much of the research work presented in this book was possible because of the financial support from the Department of Sociology, University of Uppsala (a doctoral fellowship); the Swedish Council for Planning and Coordination of Research (FRN) funding a research project on organ transplantation; Law Foundation (Rättsfonden) (a grant); and the Selma Andersen Fund at Uppsala University (a post-doctoral fellowship).

Nora Machado
Uppsala, 1998

Abbreviations

BrB:	Criminal Code (*Brottsbalken*)
HBP:	Human body part
ICU:	Intensive care unit
MF:	Code of Statutes (ordinances and guidelines) for the Medical Services published by the National Board of Health. Since 1976, the heading Mf is replaced by SOSFS (M) (*Medicinal Författning*)
NICU:	Neurological intensive care unit
ONT:	Organization Nacional de Transplantes (de España)
OPO:	Organ procurement organisation
OR:	Operation room
OTC:	Organisational Theory of Cognitive Balance
OTS:	Organ transplantation system
Proposition:	Legislative Proposals (*Proposition*). The endorsement that the Administration presents to the Parliament in the process of promulgation of a law
RF:	Swedish Constitutional Act (*Regeringsformen*). One of the fundamental acts of the Constitution that comprise the laws relating to the protection of the individual vis à vis the state (infringement of the individual right by state organs). Thus it aims to guarantee the safety and security of the citizens in the society
UAS:	Uppsala University Hospital
UNOS:	United Network for Organ Sharing

1 Introduction

The history of transplantation is, above all, a story of mythology, human fantasy, and innovation. Attempts at transplantation had been made for hundreds of years but typically resulted in death. The modern beginning of transplantation is the successful transfusion of blood. By the turn of the century, differences in human blood groups had been discovered, greatly reducing the risks of transfusions. Various attempts at solid organ transplantation were made in the first half of the century: a human kidney in Kiev in 1933, without success, and later at other medical centres in the 1940s and early 1950s, without greater success (although the physicians involved typically considered a "success" any survival for few hours or for a few days).

In 1954 Joseph E. Murray and associates successfully transplanted a kidney from one identical twin to another. During the remainder of the 1950s and throughout the 1960s, kidney transplantation increased in frequency. Organs came either from living relatives or non-heart-beating cadavers: however the cadaver kidney results were initially not as successful as those from genetically related living donors. Subsequently, not only kidney but heart transplantation (the first carried out by Christiaan Barnard in 1967) as well as other types of transplantation accelerated, particularly as knowledge about immunological defence mechanisms and ways of countering or neutralising them were developed.

Organ transplantation is today a well-established clinical treatment and part of the specialised surgical services in many hospitals in the world. The rate of successful organ replacements is quite high, particularly for kidneys, but also for the replacement of hearts, whole or parts of pancreas and livers. Today, a major development is ongoing experiments with animal grafts and genetic manipulation of animals to make their organs more compatible with human recipients.

Housing Organ Transplantation's Social Impact

Already from its outset, organ transplantation surgery was a dramatic offspring of modern heroic medicine. It promised to be a surgical panacea that would extend the life of many chronically ill and end-stage patients.

Figure 1. Usable organs and tissue from a single corpse

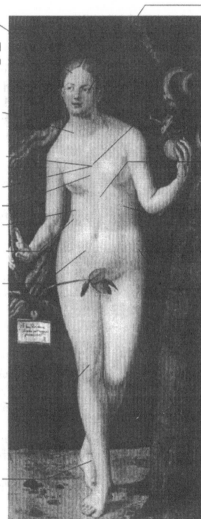

Brain tissue

1 jaw bone for facial reconstruction

Bone marrow to treat leukaemia and other diseases

4 separate valves

1 heart

2 lungs

1 liver

2 kidneys

Small and large intestines

206 separate bones, including long bones of the arms and legs for use in limb reconstruction and ribs used in spinal fusion and facial repair

About 27 ligaments and cartilage used in rebuilding ankles, knee, hips, elbows and shoulder joints

2 corneas: to restore sight

2 each of the inner ear, the hammer, anvil and stirrup: to ameliorate some forms of deafness

1 heart pericardium (can be used to cover the brain after surgery)

1 stomach (transplanted experimentally without much success)

1 pancreas (can restore insulin production in diabetes)

2 hip joints

Over 600.000 miles of blood vessels, mostly veins that can be transplanted to re-route blood around blockages

Approximately 20 square feet of skin which can be used as temporary covering for burn injuries

In more than one sense organ transplantation suited popular visions of a science that in a foreseeable future would make it possible to establish human colonies on the moon and to extend human life almost indefinitely.

The expansion and development of organ transplantation as regular procedures in health care services has had an impact beyond the clinic. It has affected the legal, organisational and cultural conditions for the access, use and transfer of body parts for therapeutic and research purposes. In particular, the demand for biological tissue and organs in health care services makes the attitudes and conceptions of people regarding the disposal of their own remains and their next of kin's bodies after death – otherwise a private or family affair – a matter of health care policies and legislation. These concerns are of critical importance in how transplantation systems operate and are understood and accepted by the people participating in or affected by them. In this regard the implementation of this biotechnology – and related policy and legal formulations – is consequential for social understandings about bodies, death and giving, or the relation between a person's rights and the collective rights with respect to her body and its parts.

An unintended consequence of these developments has been the revival of philosophical and ethical issues concerning the body, consciousness, existence and identity in the context of contemporary high technology medicine. Along these lines, Featherstone et al. (1991) points out, the impact of scientific high technology in medicine has raised difficult philosophical and ethical problems: for example, who ultimately has legal ownership of parts of human bodies? What is the role of the state in protecting the patients from unwarranted or unethical medical action? What are the professional and sociocultural risks of organ transplantation over the long run?

Symbolically, the process of organ transfer as such conveys a powerful metaphor. The process that takes place in a transplantation is a true metamorphosis – the transformation of a deceased's body part into a suitable biomedical implant – where the meaning of a body part gets redefined along the way. This transformation from *deceased somebody* into graft organ implies the crossing of many boundaries, not only physiological, but also cultural, legal and ethical ones. Such transgression of borders in many senses of the term is noted by Braun and Joerges (1993:1):

> The building up and the dynamics of European and the transborder organ transplant systems can hardly be understood without taking into account the blurring of categories between body and machine, between gift and commodity, between individual and collective ownership, between moral duty and abomination, between life and death.

The organisation and management of this alchemy of transforming the dead into "living" organs is institutionalised in an organ transplantation system. This process configures an axis of polarities, a social process, stretching between a braindead donor at one extreme and an organ receiver at the other. This process is characterised by particular social definitions and social rule systems associated with such socially defined states as "alive", "braindead", "patient", "organ donor" etc. The social rules applying to the different states indicate what is the correct and appropriate treatment towards a person in one or another state, whether a dead person or a living patient with different degree of life or living. A "deceased" is not the same as a "cadaver" because while the first term implies a set of social relations denoting a former person – an identifiable dead someone who has been part of a social relations network – the second term denotes an object with medical or biological connotations rather than social aspects. The deceased suggests a dead person, but still a person who has been part of a sociocultural context. The deceased still has a name, relatives, testament, property. The corpse as a dead body has already lost most of its social and subjective aspects. It is a decontextualised body, an object in a certain sense, (for which the notion of human agency is completely absent). While the body of a deceased is only a remains but still a sacred one, the cadaver is not, and, as such, this term is used for humans as well as animals, implying that the disconnection with human society is complete, thus becoming a part of the "natural world".[1]

Clearly, the use of human biological material has enormous potential due to the possibilities it opens for the cure of several debilitating and end-stage diseases (see figure 1). A transplant industry based upon foetal-tissue technology promises to dwarf the present level of organ transplantation. According to a US estimate, "foetal cell implants have the potential to offer relief to several million Americans, including one million with Parkinson's disease, 2.5 million to three million suffering from Alzheimer's disease, 25000 with Huntington's disease, 400,000 stroke victims, 5.8 million diabetics, and several hundred thousand people with spinal cord injuries" (Thorne, 1987). The prospect of a technical-medical development based on massive utilisation of human biological material does not belong to science fiction any longer.

Solid organ transplantation (heart, kidneys, liver, lungs, pancreas) offers the most dramatic life-saving dimension, and the greatest publicity to transplantation practice. It promotes the idea that the medical profession can through heroic measures overcome death and prolong life. Human tissue transplants are for the most part life-enhancing rather than life saving, but solid organ transplants are more dramatic and newsworthy than life-enhancing tissue implants. Organ and tissue transplantation, linked closely to the use of high technology and science, has come to be regarded by much of the public as epitomising the advancement and development of society – there is an aura of excitement, a wonderment associated with the transplantation of solid organs (O'Neill, 1996:5-6).

The Sociology of Organ Transplantation

How can sociology be applied to the study, and contribute to the understanding, of transplantation processes and systems? An organ transplantation system (hereafter OTS) can be systematically investigated in terms of, among other things, its complex social organisation, its legal and administrative aspects, the involvement of multiple professions, and the management of organ exchange in national and international networks. The OTS is characterised by precise co-ordination and tight coupling of many types of actors and activities using complex sophisticated technologies. The social processes, organisational and professional features, legal and cultural aspects of the OTS are among the possible important topics for sociological research. The impact of such technological development on social life is another potential area of sociological research. Cultural factors are also worthy of study in that they shape the ways in which people view and react to transplantation – not least the use of human body parts – and affect its operation and development. A number of interesting research questions can be imagined in any broad consideration of organ transplantation. This can be done with different approaches or perspectives depending on the interests of the researcher.

As of today, there are few sociological studies of organ transplantation. In the USA, Renée Fox and Roberta Simmons with her associates are undoubtedly the leading sociologists working in this field. Fox's research has a strong cultural orientation that can be characterised as a "thick" analytic and interpretative description of important themes in the sociology of medicine and therapeutic innovation: the medical profession, human experimentation, medical technology, dialysis and transplantation. It concerns the cluster of surgical, medical and technological means for treating certain end-stage diseases that occupy a central and consistent place within medicine and the public imagination

(Fox, 1959; 1988; 1989, etc.). *The Courage to Fail* (Fox and Sweazy, 1974) is one of the pioneering sociological studies in research on transplantation and dialysis. Over a period of four years, the authors collected data through field research (participant observation, face-to-face interviews, analysis of documents, etc.) in transplant and dialysis centres located in several regions of the USA. Their work presents a broad tapestry of the dilemmas and ambivalence associated with clinical medical research, and also attends to the impact that kidney transplantation has had on physicians as well as recipients, donors and their families.

For example, the development of new technologies such as heart and kidney transplantation and dialysis created for the physicians involved new types of decision problems and new ethical dilemmas. There were no established norms and guidelines to direct them, to help them make difficult moral choices, for instance, in determining who should get access to the scarce life-giving techniques. Over time, physicians developed new criteria for making difficult life-and-death decisions. These technological developments have not been unproblematic or an unmitigated good. One of Fox's major ideas (Fox, 1984) is that the development of modern medical technologies not only creates new types of dilemmas and types of decision problems, but has brought forth circumstances where the institutionalised strategies of "save-life-at-all costs" and "aggressive intervention" are considered less and less appropriate. Fox sees a contemporary trend toward a new medical approach oriented less to the sanctity of life and "save-life-at-all-costs" and more to the "quality of life". This is reflected in professional and popular movements for "death with dignity", and "the right to die". This trend reflects, in her view, a major shift in cultural assumptions about health and illness in the USA (see also Anspach, 1993:41).[2]

In Europe, Bernward Joerges and his group at the Wissenschaftszentrum Berlin have studied organ transplantation from the perspective of large-scale technical systems with networked operations that are not only technical but non-technical in character. (Joerges, 1988; Joerges and Braun, 1990).[3] Such a system consists of a variety of different parts or subsystems: organisational, professional, technical units, hospitals and transplantation centres in different countries. It entails a highly complex organisation. Their approach examines, in part, the interlining features of complex, technical systems and, in part, the boundaries and limits between a large-scale technical system such as organ transplantation and its environment.[4]

One aspect of "large-scale" is the high dispersion, both temporally and spatially (specifically, transborder or international), and the *interdependent technical heterogeneity.* Such systems link a wide spectrum of *varied* technologies and occupational and professional groups – not only medical but also non-medical. Joerges and his colleagues stress that because organ transplantation systems are, both spatially and functionally, widely dispersed, they require a high degree of standardisation and *compatibilisation* of the organisation, the communication systems, and exchange relationships. Systems such as OTS – they also refer to hazardous waste disposal – are considered "infrastructural service systems". They are science-intensive but also highly dependent on public acceptance and legitimisation.

Transplantation has not simply been a surgical technique. It is closely associated with the expansion of immunological and genetic research (Braun, 1994). In contrast to many other large technical systems, "affected parties" play an important role, that is recipients and their relatives, as well as donors on whom the system is greatly dependent for a strategic resource (Braun, 1994:11). The functioning of transplantation systems is constrained by the scarcity of organs, and there has been a growing gap between transplant demand and supply. For instance, in Germany, as elsewhere, the number of grafts obtained has grown continually over the past twenty years but the chance of a person on a waiting list receiving a transplant has dropped in relative terms (Braun, 1994:15). Braun correctly points out that the supply of organs for transplantation depends primarily on the medical definition of death, the number of actual deaths fitting the definition, the commitment of physicians to organ transplantation surgery, and the willingness of the population to donate organs or to support legislation providing ready access. Also, as with other current medical biotechniques, it is to a large extent embedded in the higher-level organisation of medical services, but its functioning depends on broader infrastructural, structural and "transborder" conditions (Braun and Joerges, 1993).

The organisation of organ transplantation systems OTS is not only a large scale system (Joerges, 1993) but entails tightly-coupled processes of organ harvesting, organ extraction, and organ implantation as well as recipient follow-up (Cabrer et al., 1992).[5] The nature of the technical components and the mode of their integration with social components in given organisations has a decisive influence on an OTS's performance and system dynamics. In this perspective, technologies, or more generally technical artefacts, are not merely potential determinants of social relations, not merely potential products of socially regulated human activity (Winner, 1977:14). Rather, they are integral components of social systems, and as such can be objects of sociological analysis (Mayntz, 1989).[6] The sociotechnical character of OTS entails the interaction of several medical professions, and advanced medical skills and technology – such as standardised surgical techniques, appropriate equipment (for example dialysis or heart-lung machines), permanent access to support facilities (such as operation theatres, intensive care units and typing laboratories to analyse the suitability of the organs and organ-recipient matching), pharmaceuticals (essential to immunosuppression, and organ preservation).

Moreover – as in few other medical fields – organ transplantation routines are highly dependent on extra-medical technical infrastructure, in particular communication and transportation networks (mainly by road and air). This infrastructure, ranging from energy and water supply, national communication networks etc. is simply utilised by OTS agents. However, the functioning of the OTS is highly dependent of the operation and quality of these systems. Braun and Joerges (1993:14) stress the importance of the extra-medical infrastructure:

> When due to a software error, the AT&T (telephone) network broke down in 1990, transplantation activities largely came to a halt in the US. Participating hospitals could no longer be co-ordinated, and it became impossible to locate relatives of deceased patients for obtaining organ donations.

Infrastructural conditions act as constraints on, and supports to, the functioning of organ transplantation systems. Even apparently marginal phenomena such as traffic accidents play a role in organ supply. In many countries, victims of accidents (particularly motorcycle accidents) with their characteristic head traumas, are an important source of organ donors (these are relatively young, healthy sources). Geographical factors such as the size of an organ harvesting region coupled to the transportation and communications available to the local transplantation centre, tend to affect the pattern of, for example, a heart transplantation (the optimal preservation time of a graft heart should not exceed four hours; this problem does not particularly affect geographically small European countries, but in a geographically dispersed country such as Sweden, the time needed to fly the length of the country at 800 km/h is 2.37 hours, to which must be added other moments in the transportation process not considered in the calculation; this leaves a short time marginal for implantation).

Problems with the technical infrastructural support in less industrialised countries seriously constrain effective organ transplantation. For example in India, organ transplantations are largely accomplished with living donors, since the supply of cadaveric organ donors is very low due to inadequate organisational and technical infrastructures (Slapak, 1987:18). More generally, some countries adopt these techniques without the necessary legal and cultural preparatory measures to support, for example, a "culturally accepted and politically safeguarded donor system", with the result that these countries depend on international organ supply (Braun and Joerges, 1993:26).

Another important characteristic of the OTS is, as mentioned earlier, its "transborder" character. Locally based organ transplantation organisations today are participants in a transborder organ transplantation system (Braun and Joerges, 1993). The transborder requirements of OTS means that the various health care systems participating harmonise not only technically, but also professionally, and in legal, economic or even moral respects. Much of the compatibilisation of administrative and professional formats in OTS is highly technical, for instance in the application of standard tests for tissue typification and the exchange of computerised data. The communication system PIONEER, introduced by the Eurotransplant organisation in the late 1980s in order to link all relevant transplant organisations – medical as well as non-medical – in the participating countries, plays a key role in these standardisation processes. PIONEER links on-line 38 transplantation centres and 41 typification laboratories in five Eurotransplant member countries (Germany, Austria, Belgium, Netherlands and Luxembourg) into Eurotransplant's central mainframe in Leiden. It stores 100,000 immunological patient profiles, transplantation relevant data of potential recipients (state of health, degree of urgency, treating hospital, and so forth). Whenever a donor organ becomes available, PIONEER is to initiate the computer-controlled selection of suitable recipient and, most important, to cross-check regional waiting lists and Eurotransplant's comprehensive lists of patients awaiting transplants (Braun and Joerges, 1993:9).

The interlinkage of trans-local, trans-regional and trans-national structures, consequently results in an organisation that is spatially and functionally dispersed, with high levels of standardisation at technical and organisational and even cultural levels. An example of this can be found in the broad international implementation of common classifications systems including that defining death. The latter not only facilitates the development of organ transplantation at national levels but also at international levels.

However significant the sociotechnical demands and transborder character of OTS are, the immediate social environment of any OTS plays a major role. Sociocultural factors such as religious beliefs (Faltin et al., 1992), ethnic patterns relating to death (Callender et al., 1982), social obligations (Faltin et al. 1992), differences in education and income in the population, etc., significantly affect organ donation patterns and the potentialities of organ transplantation. Cultural factors at national levels play an important role, explaining, for example, why organ transplantation was held back many years in Japan due to popular resistance to the legislation of brain death-death criteria (Ishibashi, 1992). This apparently relates to their particular conception of death as a process in Japanese traditions (according to Lock and Honde "it takes a total of 32 years for a deceased family member to fully merge with the community of spirits and become an ancestor" (1990:110)).

Marked gender, educational, ethnic and religious cleavages in populations seem to generate conflicts about and opposition to organ harvesting, opposition that eventually undermines public trust in medical care. For example, in a multiethnic society like Singapore, it is not surprising that the Human Organ Transplants Act (1987) establishes that organs can be extracted after a person's accidental death, unless the deceased has previously declared otherwise; the Act does not, however, apply to the Muslim population (rather they must sign donor cards when they wish their organs to be extracted) (Rasheed, 1992). Heterogeneous social conditions seem to increase ethical concerns and political issues about organ transplantation. Furthermore, because transplantation entails expensive procedures, its availability is highly restricted. In most countries, the access of citizens to specialised medical services such as organ transplantation depends either on the allocation of financial resources in the health care services, or to the patient's ability to pay for the operation themselves. In India, the financial burden of transplantation surgery is frequently ten times the average annual income *per capita*, and the cost of *post-transplant* immunosuppression for a single patient may be four times the average annual income per capita; at the same time, the life expectancy of a patient receiving chronic hemodialysis in India is limited to 6 months (Slapak, 1987:17).

In general terms – notwithstanding the particular religious beliefs or levels of education – family refusal to consent to organ donation of a deceased relative, as well as physicians' failure to refer potential donors, are often mentioned as the main causes of the endemic and generalised organ shortage (Levey et al., 1986). Lack of clarity about brain death, uncertainty about the proper treatment of the dead, fear of institutional abuse, suspicion of unfairness in organ allocation in the population, are common themes regarding donation refusals (Hardie et al.., 1992; Cantarovitch et al.., 1989). These are themes that in spite of the clinical standardisation of transplantation surgery reflect the concerns the practice still awakes in many societies and groups within societies around the "right" treatment of the bodies of the dead. More than 30 years after the initial successes of the 1960s, the problematic character of organ transplantation remains. As Rettig (1987:191-192) rightfully points out:

> Organ transplantation.encompasses not one but several controversies. New developments continuously extend clinical capabilities and stretch fundamental community norms. These developments include new definitions of when death occurs, the legal and ethical bases for organ donation, the ownership of organs and bodies, the relation of the state to the individual, and the role of governments and markets.

In sum, organ transplantation can be analysed from a number of different perspectives: the study of public attitudes toward a new technological development, changing concepts of life, death and the body, socialpsychological reactions to death and dying; the politics of death and the body, among others. This book focuses on several key organisational features as well as legal and ethical aspects of organ transplantation. Organ acquisition, transplantation and relevant follow-up processes are organised and regulated within formal organisations and professional networks. They entail specific activities, techniques, and technologies with a variety of actors involved and guided and regulated by particular systems of rules, including laws, administrative regulations, medical and other professional norms as well as everyday-life norms. In this complex web there are multiple incongruencies, tensions and conflicts. Developing new techniques and technologies in relation to the use of human bodies and dealing with the dead is not, therefore, straightforward.

Human biological material such as necroorgans and tissue are an increasingly valuable and scarce good. The ways in which this "valuable material" should be defined, procured, utilised and distributed is a matter of controversy. Critical ethical, legal and cultural questions are evoked by the application of transplantation surgery: the regulation of body part extraction and use; ambiguous feelings of next-of-kin and medical personnel related to braindead donors; ethical dilemmas associated with organ request and the selection and prioritisation of organ recipients, among others.

In spite of major educational campaigns and the widespread public support for organ donation indicated by public opinion surveys, people appear to have reservations about writing donor cards or allowing the extraction of organs from deceased relatives. Ambivalence is expressed by relatives of the potential donors and even by health care personnel involved in transplantation procedures. These arise in part in connection with the ambiguity of life-and-death boundaries that are embodied in the concept of "braindead donor".

2 Key Processes in Organ Transplantation

The aim of this chapter is to identify and schematise several of the key social processes involved in transplantation. The chapter goes on to develop process models of kidney transplantation in a major transplantation centre in Sweden, showing the path of the organs from donors to patients, the actors involved and several of the important rule complexes governing their decisions and actions.[7]

A Transplantation Story

A organ transplantation may start with a cerebral haemorrhage or perhaps a motorcycle accident. The victim, now a patient, will be quickly transported to the emergency unit of the nearest hospital. Here, the physician on duty will examine the patient and give the first clinical assessment about her neurological state on a scale from 1 (fully awake) to 8 (totally unconscious). Already at the midpoint of the scale, the likelihood of severe brain damage is significant.

When brain damage is feared or has already taken place, the patient will be quickly transported to the neurological intensive care unit of the hospital, if no other physical traumas require prior surgical intervention. In a deep state of unconsciousness, the patient will be attached to life-supoport (a ventilator to assist respiration). She will be now examined to determine the extent of the cerebral damage. Several clinical tests and perhaps a brain scan will be performed. If the tests show no signs of cerebral activity a total and irreversible brain damage is presumed. After confirmatory tests, if the results are similar, the death of the patient – as brain death[8] – will be verified.

The family or the next-of-kin of the newly braindead patient is now to be informed by the attending physician that death has been certified. Most often they will also be informed about "organ donation". Sometimes they will have to decide whether or not to allow an organ donation, but commonly they will be asked what their relative would have eventually wanted to be done with her body. If the family authorises the extraction of one or several organs, the braindead patient will be maintained in a ventilator until the organ extraction can be carried out.

At this stage the "transplantation co-ordinator" of the hospital or transplantation centre, usually a nurse, is already informed about the available donor and will gather information on the case and order some tests to determine if the deceased is a suitable donor (i.e. the cause of death, the condition of the organs, eventual diseases etc., and to determine blood group, tissue type, etc. in order to find compatible recipients). Also, she will instruct the nurses of the intensive care unit how to proceed in order to maintain the body until the extraction can be co-ordinated.

The transplantation co-ordinator would already have alerted the surgeons on duty that a "donor call" has been received. This means that an organ extraction (and a transplantation) can be expected in the hours ahead. Samples of blood and tissue of the deceased will be sent to the laboratory of the hospital or the transplantation centre. When the first results of the tests arrive, the lists of patients waiting for organs in the region covered by the transplantation centre will be reviewed; but the national lists will also be checked to see what organs are needed, or if there is a priority case that should receive some particular organ first (see Chapter 4).

Those to be selected as organ receivers will be finally chosen some hours later or the next day, when the results of compatibility tests between the available parts and the possible candidates are ready. Next, the selected recipients will be called to the hospital and prepared for operation.

***

Organ transplantation surgery comprises two stages, the organ extraction, and the implantation of those organs into recipients. In principle, two transplantation teams are involved in each phase, on the one hand the removal team(s), on the other the transplant team(s) that will implant those organs into recipients. The removal team(s) travels to the hospital where the donor's body is located.

***

When everything is ready, the body of the donor, still attached to the ventilator, will be taken to the operation theatre. The organs will be now extracted one by one and the ventilator disconnected. The organs are soaked in perfusion liquids and placed in cold boxes. They are now ready to be transported to transplantation centres. The body of the donor is prepared and usually transported to the pathology section of the hospital for the eventual extraction of tissue, and thereafter to the morgue of the hospital.

Parallel to the process of procuring organs are the processes of selecting recipients. For instance, a physician or clinic first proposes a patient for transplantation. This is typically somebody whose survival (or quality of life) requires an organ. A related criterion concerns the urgency of the transplantation. Potential recipients of, for instance, a kidney, may be maintained on dialysis while waiting. But the urgency for patients in need of heart, lung, and liver organs may be precisely because of their rapidly deteriorating condition. But the patient may be judged to be far too sick to undergo a transplantation; for example, a patient in Uppsala in need of a heart transplant was sent to Gothenburg to await a heart transplant (Gothenburg's transplant centre is the only one regularly conducting heart transplantation in Sweden). But his condition worsened (suffering from renal and liver problems he was judged unable to sustain a transplant operation). He was returned to Uppsala where he subsequently died.

In the case of kidneys, a transplantation centre has a waiting list of potential recipients. One or both kidneys are allocated among the patients on the waiting list of the region according to: (1) blood type compatibility, (2) tissue type compatibility between patient and organ, (3) regional priority, (4) time on the waiting list, (5) state of the health of the potential recipients at the moment of the organ arrival, (6) special emergency or contingency to take into account in the prioritisation of a particular patient, e.g. characteristics of the patient and the advantages or disadvantages that may entail for future success. The selection of the patient is discussed within the transplantation team, together with the head nurse of the unit and a social assistant (who has the function of assisting the patients with social, financial or logistical problems associated with their stay at the hospital or their disease).

Transplantation Process and Organisation

Transplantation is the therapeutic replacement of diseased organs and tissues by means of healthy ones. Specifically, it is the transfer of organ tissue, or fluid from one human body or animal to another human body or the transfer from a living body back to itself. Organ transplantation entails a social and technical process – a network of co-operating and exchanging units, including administrative units – in which numerous actors in different roles are involved. A variety of technologies and techniques are utilised in the process. The actors involved are co-ordinated and regulated through administrative and exchange relations, to a great extent shaped and governed by particular regulations, laws, professional norms, and institutional arrangements.

The supply of organs is a decisive factor in the network. Most organs for transplantation are obtained from deceased donors. Giving the legal premises existing in most countries where transplantations are performed (where some kind of authorisation is required from the donor), the public attitude towards donation is of great importance. In most Western countries there is a general acceptance of the notion of organ donation for therapeutic purposes. A survey in the USA in 1993 showed that 85% of the population in the US support organ donation, and that almost 70% were quite willing to give their own organs after death (Gallup, 1993). Swedish surveys concerning attitudes towards donation show that up to 70% of the population expresses a willingness to donate organs after death (Gäbel and Lindskoug, 1987). However, in practice high percentages of next-of-kin refuse to allow organ donation from their deceased relatives [in approximately 40% of the cases, the relatives vetoed the donation in Sweden (Gäbel, 1992), and about 30% of the approached relatives did not give authorisation to donate the organs in the USA (Gallup, 1993)].

Organ transplantation depends to a large extent on having legitimacy in the larger society, not only in terms of authorisation and financing of particular techniques, but also in terms of gaining access to and using body parts. Regarding the use of body parts for transplantation, there are multiple cognitive frameworks and interests, different rights, obligations, authorities, and powers. Ethical, religious, and cultural dilemmas arise. A central matter is the distinction between the sacred and the profane and the boundary between them. This boundary is possibly shifting; but it also varies for the different categories of actors involved (see Chapters 5-9).

Transplantation surgery can no longer be understood as an expression of "heroic medicine" – even if an heroic dimension is also discernible and the drama of those patients whose lives or quality of life depend on a transplantation is very real. Today it works as a complex system with multiple linkages and a substantial internal dynamics.

OTS as Administrative System and Exchange Network

A part of the OTS co-ordination is organised administratively, e.g. within a major hospital, the transplantation centre where organ transplantation surgery is carried out. The actors in the organisation are organised and co-ordinated through particular institutional arrangements. The transplantation system is thus imbedded in larger systems, such as the health care system and, in a wider frame, legal, cultural, and historic frameworks. Among the basic requirements for the functioning of a transplantation system are: (1) access to a pool of organs (i.e. potential donors prepared to donate); (2) skilled medical professionals; (3) access to support technology such as typing laboratories, dialysis, immunosuppressives, etc.; (4) communication networks; (5) transportation networks. The OTS organisation enables the mobilisation and co-ordination in transplantation processes of special expertise (medical and other personnel), resources, technologies (drugs, laboratories, transport), and diverse "production structures" (potential donors and selected patients defined as potential organ receivers). In short, the OTS consists of various structures linking, regulating, and monitoring a complex, advanced sociotechnical system.[9]

The OTS is, however, not only an administrative system mobilising and co-ordinating resources but also an extensive exchange network which shares information and organs. This co-ordination is organised through networks of organisations without authority over one another, but nonetheless adhering to common rules, for example rules giving priority to particular types of recipients and thus motivating a particular allocation of organs. The exchange networks originated with the need to increase the local pool of donated kidneys through organ exchange. Through the network professionals exchange information and monitor the data lists of patients waiting for organs, with the purpose of finding a match as close as possible between the tissue-type of the recipients and the donated organs. Such matching is believed to increase the likelihood of successful transplantation. Also the networks spread information about potential donors (organs) with particular characteristics that can be matched with patients with certain antigen profiles waiting for organs.

Common arrangements regarding exchange rules for organs such as kidneys are that when an available kidney has a high compatibility with an already high immunised patient on a waiting list on a more global level, one may bypass the local waiting list and remit the organ to that particular patient.[10] In this way, one of the two kidneys obtained is remitted to the sensitised patient while the other is transplanted at the local centre. Concerning scarcer organs such as hearts, lungs and livers there is a waiting list common to all members of the network, with special priorities for urgent cases at national or regional levels.

These organ and information sharing networks often cover more than one country – linking its transplantation centres to an international sphere, e.g. Scandiatransplant in Scandinavia and Eurotransplant for Germany, Austria and the Benelux countries. The "internationalisation" of national medical systems is particularly noteworthy, given earlier patterns of institutional closure in hospital or national regional networks – except for medical research and scientific exchange. There are several explanations for this extension of the system into a large-scale infrastructural order (these do not exclude one another):

- The larger exchange network implies increasing access to a larger variety and population of organs and potential recipients with particular profiles (antigen profiles) that increases the likelihood of effective matching. [11]

- The exchange network allows for a more efficient use of available organs in that temporary surpluses (which, given limited storage possibilities, implies organ wastage) will be effectively used rather than thrown away. Large, stable pools of organs through extensive exchange networks buffer or smooth out local supply/demand imbalances. A temporary local surplus of organs can be distributed elsewhere; or a temporary local shortage can be covered by organs from other regions or nations.

The exchange of organs between centres organised through the organ sharing network is co-ordinated according to specific rules (i.e. giving priority to particular types of recipients and thus motivating particular allocation of organs). The exchange rules of the organ sharing network may clash with the allocation rules of the local centre (for example, concerning emergency cases where a patient may die of liver or pancreas failure if a transplantation is not carried out immediately even with a low compatibility organ (that by organ network rules should be allocated elsewhere). Thus, there may arise structural tensions between the responsibility of the local network to its patients and the rules of the non-local network.[12] Infraction of these rules is informally disapproved (no particular administrative or legal sanction is established for a centre breaking, e.g., exchange rules).[13]

Particular Sociotechnical Characteristics of the OTS

The development of immunosuppression therapy has been crucial in preventing organ rejection, and is thus a central factor in making the expansion of transplantation surgery technically possible. Today, cyclosporine combined with other immunosuppressants is the usual formula utilised in therapy.

The transportation and storage of organs is an important technical factor in the process of organ extraction, distribution and allocation. The cooperation and exchange between transplantation centres at regional, national and international levels relies on the adequate transportation of blood samples, organs, and personnel and patients around the region, and also on an operative communication system. The survival time of the organs outside of the donor's body is quite short, even if better methods of organ preservation have been developed. Thus, the effectiveness of organ transport and maintenance is not a negligible factor in the success rate and development of organ transplantation.

Maintenance of organs for transplantation requires an adequate cold environment for the organ (cold solutions in thermal boxes) during the transport and eventual storage or ischemic time (the time that the organs are outside the donor's body and consequently without blood circulation). The development of better storage techniques has made it possible to maintain organs in good condition for longer periods and to transport the organs over greater distances. This is quite important since increased time marginals decreases the risk of organ wastage.[14] The ischemic time varies for each organ (generally accepted figures are shown in the table below). The mortality risk for a heart recipient increases by 6% for each hour that the organ is without blood circulation.

Table 1. Ischemic times (maxima) for different organs

Heart	up to 5 hours
Heart-Lung	up to 5 hours
Lung	up to 6 hours
Liver	up to 34 hours
Pancreas	up to 20 hours
Kidney	up to 72 hours
Bone Marrow	varies with the individual program
Corneas	up to 10 days
Heart Valves	5 years or more
Skin	5 years or more
Bone	5 years or more

Source: National Kidney Foundation, 1996, US; United Network for Organ Sharing, 1996.

A network of transplantation centres typically shares a common database with a list of patients waiting on the respective lists and relevant information about their medical status (tissue type, blood group, etc.). Otherwise, "organ calls" are sent to other centres by fax or telephone. Also, most of the patients on the waiting lists are equipped with pagers so they can be contacted by the transplantation centre at any time, whenever an organ becomes available. Characteristic of this type of arrangement is the "tight coupling" – that is the limited technical, time and geographical operative marginals – requiring a precise co-ordination of many types of activities and actors using complex, advanced technologies.

Systemic Models of Organ Transplantation Processes

The transplantation of organs entails then a complex organisation, that engages various health professionals with different skills and roles, acting in institutions or settings connected to each other and constituting networks of organ and information exchange. The activities performed by the professionals and the institutional settings where they operate are governed by rules and principles of organisation that define, order, limit and make possible these activities. The rule complex includes not only formalised rules but also the informal, unwritten and implicit ones, such as moral codes, administrative organisation principles etc. (Burns and Flam. 1987). Professional groups are organised and co-ordinated through specific organisations such as hospitals, embedded in larger institutional and cultural settings. The latter provide the structure of rules and meta-rules (e.g. laws, government policies, professional norms and standards, ethical values, etc.), and, in general, the cultural-societal frame within which the transplantation system operates. Included in the larger cultural-societal frame are specific laws and regulations steering and constraining transplantation activities, such as the Transplants Act in Sweden.

The Swedish OTS

The Swedish OTS is embedded in a larger system, the Swedish Health Care organisation, and, in a wider perspective, infrastructural, legal and socio-cultural settings. Basically, the particular requirements of the organisation are a sizeable pool of donors/organs for transplantation, skilled professionals (surgeons and other specialists), technical means (such as appropriate laboratories, drugs such as immunosuppresors etc.), and communication and transportation networks.

The Organisational Environment: The Swedish Health Care System

The Swedish health care organisation is largely the result of centralised planning. The more specialised and technically advanced medical activities are, the more they are part of a national plan. The system allows for private practitioners and a few, relatively small, private hospitals, and these are not authorised to perform transplants.

Organ transplantation, as one of the more expensive and specialised medical treatments, has been subject to attempts at strict national planning and co-ordination, taking into consideration the calculated need of transplants per year and the available resources; this has been the responsibility of the National Board of Health Care and the Association of County Councils. Sweden is divided into health care areas at the local, regional and national levels, and public authorities are responsible for the provision of public health care services to the population at each level. Every public hospital has its own area of responsibility and is in a sense a monopoly.[15]

Public health insurance covers the whole population and is financed regionally by taxes levied by the *Landsting* (counties). Medical services are paid by the county where the individual lives, and since health care is supposed to be equally available in all counties and few counties provide transplantation services, organ transplantation surgery is in most cases bought and sold between the counties. All patients are eligible for transplantation independently of the county where they live, and the home county must pay the cost of the surgery. There are regulatory systems to ensure that services and costs are evenly distributed, such as formal agreements between counties.

The Organisational Goal: The Organ Recipients

According to official estimates the need for kidneys for transplantation in Sweden is over 400 per year. The supply of organs today does not cover the demand (see Table 2). The waiting time for patients is between 6 months and two years. In order for the organisation to achieve a high level of efficiency, given the scarcity of organs, the selection and prioritisation of patients is important. The choice of recipients (or the correct allocation of organs) is regarded as one of the important factors in a successful transplantation (Banta et al., 1989:6).

The guidelines applied in the prioritisation and selection of patients for transplantation indicate some variation between centres, but the general premises are similar. These consist of a series of criteria, where the main one is a strictly medical criterion (severity and nature of organ dysfunction). There is also an efficiency criterion (related to life expectancy – e.g. patients with liver cancer), an administrative criterion (e.g. waiting time in the list), and collaterally psychosocial criteria (e.g. whether patients with alcohol-related liver cirrhosis should be offered liver transplantation).

Table 2. Renal transplantation statistics in Scandinavia

	Sweden	Finland	Norway	Denmark	Total
Million inhabitants	8.75	5.08	4.30	5.22	23.35
Number of necrodonors	104	99	65	73	341
Necrodonors PMP	11.9	19.5	15.1	14.0	14.6
Necrokidney transplantations	209	175	117	136	637
Living donor kidney transplantations	99	3	69	42	213
% living donor kidney transplantations	31.1	1.7	36.0	23.6	25.0
Kidney waiting list size December 31, 1996	433	172	116	277	998
% patients with PRA >80%	4.2	8.7	3.4	3.6	4.7
Renal transplants PMP	35.2	35.0	43.3	34.1	34.4

Figures are given by country and are summarised for Scandiatransplant in the right-hand column. PMP: per million population; PRA: panel reactive antibodies (see Chapter 4 for explanation).

Source: Scandiatransplant, 1996.

The Input: Procured Organs

The main source of organs transplanted in each centre is its own recovery area, secondly other regions in the country, thirdly the Scandinavian area (organised by Scandiatransplant), and finally Europe through the different European co-ordination centres. This order operates especially for kidneys, but also functions for other organs as well as for highly sensitised patients that require a high degree of tissue compatibility.

Key actors in the process of organ procurement are the physicians at the ICUs of the regional hospital and in the hospitals of the harvesting region. There is no obligation for health personnel to request organs, but a commission appointed by the Swedish government to prepare the basis for legislative changes on transplantations suggested that the organ request should be regularly made by the personnel in charge of the case, i.e., the physician (SOU 1998:98).

The terms of organ procurement are regulated in Sweden by the Transplants Act. This law regulates the conditions for living and necro forms of organ procurement and is based on a presumption of consent (see Chapter 9). In Sweden, authorisation for organ extraction is given in 70-80% of cases (Groth,1989:4591), even if more recent studies suggest that authorisation rates have decreased considerably (Gäbel, 1992).

The Levels of the OTS

In the structure of the Swedish Organ Transplantation System, four levels of organisation/co-ordination can be distinguished. The first level is the transplantation centre located at the hospital where the unit that carries out the transplantations is situated. This level comprises the transplantation unit, and all other units in the hospitals that are engaged in the organ transplantation process. This includes the intensive care units (ICU), in particular the neurological intensive care unit (NICU), the operating rooms, anesthesiology, laboratories, surgical and medical wards as well as non-medical units such as hospital transport etc.

The second level of the Swedish OTS is the regional level. Sweden has four regions and 5 transplantation centres: Huddinge Hospital in Stockholm; Malmö General Hospital and Lund Hospital;[16] Uppsala University Hospital; and Sahlgrenska Hospital in Gothenburg. Each transplantation centre has a geographical region assigned to it where less specialised hospitals responsible for regional and primary care are located. The assigned region functions as an organ harvesting area, and receives the services of the transplantation centre, with the exception of heart-lung transplantations.[17] The latter are largely restricted to the transplantation centre at Gothenburg that, for this reason, has a national harvesting area for hearts and lungs.

The third level of the OTS is the Swedish/Nordic cooperation level. This level includes the four Swedish transplantation centres, one in Norway, four in Denmark and one in Finland. These centres co-operate forming an organ sharing network, Scandiatransplant.[18] The main purpose of this network organisation is the exchange of organs and information to allow better organ-receiver matching[19] but also to enable professional cooperation between centres in the form of transplantation surgeons performing operations at other hospitals in the organisation.

The fourth level is the West European level. In Western Europe there are several organ-sharing networks. This level of cooperation concerns in general other organs than kidneys. Organs are shared when there is an urgent call for an organ that is not available in the home country. From the Swedish perspective the most important one is Eurotransplant.

This cooperation at different levels enables better tissue match between graft and patient, and concerns especially kidneys and pancreas. Regarding other organs, e.g. hearts or livers, the match only concerns adequate blood group and/or size. The more recipients to choose from the greater the likelihood of finding one that fits well with the donated organ and vice-versa,[20] or finding organs on short notice.

The Hospital Level

Here I shall focus on one of the transplantation centres, the University Hospital in Uppsala (UAS). UAS specialises in kidney transplantation but transplantation of pancreas and livers is also common. The UAS is the largest hospital of the county and one of the largest in the country (approx. 1800 beds). It provides almost all medical specialties, including kidneys and pancreas transplantation. The UAS transplantation centre was established as a separate unit in 1992. This related to the establishment of a joint cooperation program with the Stockholm transplantation region (Huddinge transplantation centre) but it is still a relatively small unit at the hospital. Previously, transplantation surgery was performed at the Department of Urology.

The other transplantation centres in the country are located at hospitals of similar size and facilities. However, their organisations differ according to several factors, the type of organs replaced, the particular organisational history of the transplantation centre, the distribution and eventual specialisation of the cooperating hospitals in the harvesting region, and naturally the internal organisation of the unit.

The activity in the transplantation unit specifically consists of the removal of organ(s) from living and necrodonors, the transplantation of the organ(s) in patients,[21] the monitoring of operated patients in the ward, the periodical follow-ups of previously transplanted patients, retransplantations, evaluation of transplant candidates, maintenance of network links with the hospitals of the region plus periodical informational and educational crusades to hospitals and nursing schools.

Most often the procurement allows for the extraction of more than one organ. These organs may be transplanted into patients in different hospitals and regions. If heart and/or lung are to be extracted, a team from the centre that will perform the transplantation (i.e. a thoracic team) performs in turn the necessary extractions.[22] Meanwhile, given the time constraints on the preservation of an organ without blood circulation (cold ischemic time), the recipient normally will be waiting at the hospital when the graft arrives. The UAS transplantation unit depends heavily on having access to technical and organisational support, and collaborates closely with several other units in the hospital in providing care and service to recipients.

Figure 2. The Transplantation Hospital: Frequently Cooperating Units

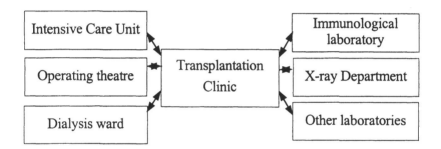

The transplantation unit needs access to adequate laboratories (for tissue matching or typing, cyto-immunological analysis, biopsies, etc.), and to an intensive care unit.[23] It also requires a capacity to provide infection therapy, equipment to treat all forms of renal insufficiency; access (and priority to access) to operation units and anesthesiology, and specialised surgeons available 24 hours a day. Also important is the availability of non-medical services such as transportation, and access to communication networks. The transplantation centre's most frequent contacts are with the dialysis ward, the operation theatres, immunology, X-ray section, and laboratories. Laboratories are particularly important because of the central role of tissue matching, profilaxis and immunosuppressive therapy in avoiding organ rejection. Of course, OTS shares the general infrastructure of the hospital (administration, access to basic hospital equipment, cleaning, repairing, etc.). Some of the medical and non-medical services to the transplantation unit can be planned or procured ahead of time. Others must be obtained on an emergency basis (e.g. tissue typing).

Intensive Care Units: The collaboration between the transplantation centre and the two intensive care units, the general intensive care unit (ICU) and the neurological ICU, are of great importance for organ recovery since all organ donors at UAS pass through one of these units.[24] It is in the ICUs that potential donors are detected and assessed, and brain death eventually determined. When the status of potential donors is determined, the transplantation centre is contacted. This is the usual starting point of the cooperation around a transplantation.

According to Swedish law (see Chapter 9), a physician in charge of a patient waiting for a transplant cannot determine the death status of a potential donor or be involved in the decision of extracting the organs. The rationale behind this clause in the Transplants Act is to avoid conflicts of interest on the part of medical practitioners and to safeguard the rights of seriously ill or dying patients, assuring that they receive the appropriate care without other considerations such as transplantation needs. Thus, assessing an individual as a potential donor and determining her death status is the responsibility of the physicians at intensive care units. The detection and referral of potential donors by the physicians in intensive units has a voluntary character. However, it is regarded as highly desirable that the medical personnel collaborate with the transplantation centre (SOU 1989:98), and they are also encouraged to do so by the centre.

When an individual's death (brain death) is determined, and if the organs are suitable for transplantation, referral is made to the transplantation unit. The latter starts the preparation for the operation and instructs the ICU personnel about any necessary procedures to assure viability of the organs. If the disposition of the deceased regarding organ donation is not known, the next of kin of the deceased are contacted to discuss an eventual donation.[25]

Usually the intensive care units can meet the needs of the transplantation unit without major alterations in their organisation or practices. However, if the care of braindead donors demands extra time in ICUs and extra personnel have to be engaged in the maintenance of the organs before the extraction, the transplantation unit reimburses the costs.[26]

The Operation Theatre: Several of the operation theatres at the UAS are organisationally integrated into a Central Operation I (OR). The surgical departments, including transplantation surgery, use the theatres on a per minute basis and pay accordingly. Since the legal requirement is that organ extraction should take place within 24 hours after the certification of death,[27] and the preservation of the organs sets strict time constraints, transplantation surgery is close to emergency surgery, and thus takes priority over non-emergency operations. This situation affects the planning of the OR, and may evoke tensions between the transplantation unit and the

OR.[28] Otherwise, in the hospital organisation, cooperation between the transplantation centre and the OR does not differ from many other cooperative linkages.

The Dialysis Unit: Many patients waiting for kidney transplants are under dialysis. Patients may need dialysis shortly before the operation in order to improve their general condition, and eventually after the transplantation. This is arranged in cooperation with the dialysis unit. The organisational impact on this unit is that dialysis scheduling may have to be re-arranged.

The Laboratories: The laboratories play a central role in the transplantation process. Their services are essential and must be readily available on short notice. The status of each potential recipient is tested approximately every three months, and new samples for compatibility tests are taken before an eventual transplantation. Concurrently, the donor is tested at the home hospital for compatibility and in order to discard cases of infectious diseases. Samples are also sent to the UAS for analysis.

The Transplantation Team: The transplantation team is technically divided into two groups that eventually can become specialised: an organ extract team and the transplant team that performs the operations on the recipient. The number of surgeons and nurses required for an organ extraction varies with the organ to extract. For example, the extraction of a kidney requires two surgeons, a transplantation co-ordinator (perfusionist) plus two operation nurses, while the extraction of a heart requires two thorax surgeons, one anesthesiologist, one operation nurse, one anesthesiology nurse and one perfusionist (*Transplantationsverksamhet for lever och hjärta*, 1988).

The Transplantation Co-ordinator: The function of a transplantation co-ordinator is above all to organise the logistics of the organ extraction and organ implantation. As shown in Figure 3, the activities of a Swedish transplantation co-ordinator are several: to give support to the personnel at the ICU concerning maintainance of the potential donor, necessary tests to be taken, etc.; to arrange the transportation of the extraction team to the hospital when the braindead donor is maintained; to assist in the organ extraction; to order from the laboratories the tissue typing, crossmatching and antibody tests; to maintain the waiting list up to date; to check with the Scandiatransplant list in case a identical match organ/receiver is found; to assist the physicians with the recipient selection, to call the chosen recipient the transplantation centre; to thank the relatives of the donor and the operation personnel in the local hospital that collaborated with the extraction; and finally to maintain contact with the mass-media and assist in the elaboration of educational and information programs about transplantation in the region.

Regional Level

Given the special expertise and the substantial resources it consumes, the transplantation of solid organs is restricted to five medical centres in Sweden, the Uppsala Academic Hospital (in Uppsala), Sahlgrenska Hospital (in Gothenburg), Huddinge Hospital (in Stockholm), Lund's Hospital (in Lund) and Malmö General Hospital (in Malmö).[29] These centres have the technical resources and the specialised staff to perform the operations.

Figure 3. The Activities of a Swedish Transplantation Co-ordinator

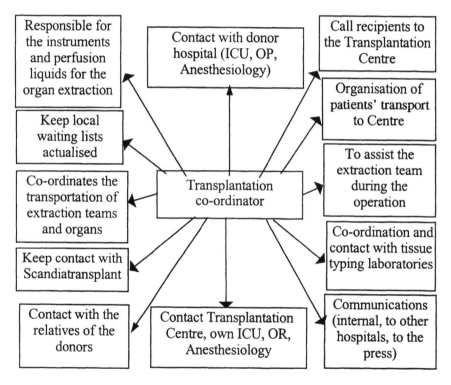

Other hospitals become, for transplantation purposes, donor hospitals – essential to the system but peripheral to the highly specialised central hospitals. The organisation at the different transplantation centres may vary due to specialisation in type of organ, and location of transplantation services at different medical departments. At the UAS, transplantation is organised as a separate unit, the centre has its own harvesting area. However, the UAS and Huddinge respective transplantation units have established a cooperation program, regarding kidney and liver transplants, sharing harvesting areas and medical services.

The transplantation centre is the hub of a network co-ordinating the acquisition of organs, the selection of recipients for the entire region, and the follow-up care of the recipients when they return to their home areas. A harvesting region usually comprises the neighbouring counties of the transplantation centre, except for northern Sweden, which is part of the Gothenburg harvesting area. For example, the regional level of the UAS transplantation centre consists of six counties including the county of Uppsala (approximately 1.7 million residents) and 22 hospitals with intensive care units as part of the regional network of organs suppliers.[30]

These hospitals have sufficient technical and professional capacity to take in patients with cerebral haemorrhages, brain tumours, head traumas etc., at least in initial stages. This level of capability is satisfied by all hospitals at the county and municipal level. Actual organ removal is carried out by a transplantation team from UAS at these hospitals. The transplantations are always performed at the UAS transplantation centre. In the region three fourths of all necroorgans come from UAS itself while a fourth comes from other hospitals in the region.[31] The patients of the region, waiting for transplantation surgery, are in a first round selected in their local hospitals and then included in the waiting list of each transplantation centre. There is a single waiting list for transplants for the whole area, and all the residents have the right of equal access to transplantation surgery.

Each county is a sort of large customer of the transplantation centre, and it covers the expenses of dialysis treatment of its residents. Each extra month on the waiting list costs around 30.000 Skr.

At every associated hospital, there is a physician at the intensive care unit responsible for the organ procurement. The contacts with the transplantation centre (detection and referral of potential donors) are made on similar premises as those with the ICUs at UAS, extra costs are paid by the UAS as transplantation costs.

When a referral from a regional hospital is received at the transplantation centre, and the consent for the organ extraction is obtained, the co-ordinator gives the instructions for the maintenance and necessary tests of the presumptive donor. Since the associated hospitals in the regions normally do not have sufficient laboratory facilities to carry out all the cross tests, and the immunological and ancillary tests (e.g. virus tests), blood samples from necrodonors are sent by plane or automobile for testing in the laboratories of the transplantation centre.

Typically, two surgeons and one transplantation co-ordinator (nurse) from the transplantation centre, travel to the associated hospital of the corresponding region, to perform the extraction. This is done by car or ambulance. If the travel distances are large, the transportation is by airplane or helicopter. For example, in the UAS region, the transportation of the team is arranged by two private transport companies, one for automobile travel and the other for helicopter and airplane travel contracted by the hospital.[32] After the extraction the team brings the organ(s) to the transplantation centre.

Table 3. Types of organ transplantation at Swedish Centres

	UAS	Huddinge	Gothenburg	Malmö/Lund
Kidney	✦	✦	✦	✦ (Malmö)
Pancreas	✦	✦	✦	✦ (Malmö)
Liver, adult	✦	✦	✦	-
Liver, child	-	-	✦	-
Heart/lung	-	-	✦	-
Heart	-	-	✦	✦ (Lund)
Lung	-	-	✦	✦ (Lund)

The patient(s) placed highest on the waiting list are forewarned about the impending transplantation and they usually come to the transplantation centre on their own. If necessary, they are transported by ambulance.

The Swedish/Nordic Level

Concerning organ exchange, the five Swedish transplantation centres in the four regions do not make up a separate organ-sharing network, since each is a member of the Nordic Transplantation Association. The cooperation between Sweden, Denmark, Norway and Finland was established in 1969, as a Nordic co-ordination agency for the exchange and distribution of kidneys for transplantation. The original aim of the co-ordination agency was (a) to provide donor kidneys that could match as closely as possible the recipient's blood and tissue type in order to increase the chances of successful transplantations; (b) to allocate kidneys that were not being used "locally" for transplantation and that otherwise would be "wasted" (see Chapter 4).

The West European Level

The co-operative network of the Swedish OTS not only includes Scandinavia but also Western Europe. The main cooperation from UAS perspective takes place with Eurotransplant and to a lesser extent with United Kingdom Transplant, France Transplant, and the other European organ-sharing networks.

The larger exchange network provides access to a greater variety and population of organs with particular profiles and exchange of information. There are, however, increased medical and organisational demands. An important reason for this is that exchange networks call for high levels of standardisation of procedures and regulations in all the involved centres – procedures and regulations that in many instances have been initially determined by national policies.

The organ-sharing cooperation network is not established on a permanent basis but is instead activated by an "urgent call for organ" from any of the Western European transplantation centres. These are urgent requests for organ of particular characteristics, that are not available at the local centre. These requests often concern other organs than kidneys. The "internationalisation" of the national medical system is particularly noteworthy, given earlier patterns of closure in hospital or national regional networks – except for research and scientific exchange. The co-ordination of organ exchange is managed by specially appointed "co-ordinators" in each transplantation centre, forming an network through the Scandinavian region and eventually with Western Europe (Nordic and European co-ordinating centres).

The Transplantation Process: Main Phases, Settings, Rules, Actors and Constraints

A transplantation process is here understood as a set of activities, organised by rule systems with various social actors involved in more or less well-defined settings. *Inputs to the process are the potential donors of human body parts (HBPs); outputs are operated patients.* There are mediating, external systems that enable effective operations (e.g., transportation systems or transnational connections for organ interchange). The actors in the system include the different specialists connected to the transplantation process, the patients, the potential donors and their families, etc.

The transplantation process can be divided into several phases including organ donation and allocation processes as well as transplantation. The multiple actors engaged in these core processes have different cognitive frameworks and interests, different social positions, rights, obligations, authorities, and powers. Two of the strategic processes where social tensions, moral dilemmas and conflicts arise are those of organ procurement and recipient selection. Several of the specific questions which the modelling methodology promises to enable us to address in specific ways are the following:

(1) *The Procurement Process*: How is organ procurement organised and carried out? Who is involved? What decisions are made in the process of procurement? How are these decisions accomplished? What legal and medical rules, cultural definitions and assessments enter into the social decisions and interactions relating to "donating organs"? What tensions or conflicts are there among participants concerning the concept of brain death, body, bodily parts?

(2) *The Organ Allocation Process*: How is recipient selection organised? Who participates in the decision? What factors are taken into consideration in the allocation decision-making: e.g., conceptions of right or proper recipients, allocation principles, medical and non-medical evaluative criteria, norms and procedures?

The two core processes of procurement and allocation involve multiple actors with different cognitive frameworks and interests, different rights and obligations, authorities, and powers. One should not view transplantation simply as a matter of some people wanting (or not wanting) to give parts and others wanting or not wanting to receive them. Ethical, religious, cultural and social dilemmas arise. Questions of the sacred and the profane and the boundary between them arise (a boundary that is probably shifting but in any case varies for different actors) (see Chapter 10). Modelling methodology enables us to organise data on complex organisational phenomena, and therefore to systematically address the types of questions indicated above. In sum, the process of transplantation is viewed here as a *social process* in which numerous actors in different roles are involved.

The transplantation process can be divided into the following main phases (see Figure 4). Each phase takes place in one or more settings governed by particular rule regimes with particular actors participating (the models are based on Swedish data, but have a family resemblance to patterns on other systems).

Settings

The different stages in the process and the corresponding decision-making and activities take place in different settings. The various settings are governed by specific rules and scopes of action.

Political-administrative decision settings: Responsibility for the organisation of the health system in general (transplantation included) rests with the Association of Swedish County Councils (ASSC) in collaboration with the National Board of Health and Welfare (NBHW). Their function is to assist the organisation and effective functioning of the system, to guarantee the quality and safety of medical care, and to ensure that the highly specialised medical care will be available to all the inhabitants of the country (Transplantationsverksamhet for lever och hjärta, 1988). At the macro-institutional level, the key actors are the ASCC and the NBHW along with representatives of the regional hospitals.

Specific organisational settings: Transplantations are primarily performed at the level of regional health care: the former is a very specialised health care service and includes highly specialised regional hospitals (i.e. in Sweden, university hospitals). A region includes several counties.

The agencies for organ exchange: A central function of the co-ordinating centres for organ exchange is to increase access to organs of the transplantation centres. The co-ordination of the information about available organs in the different sub-regions and hospitals helps to allocate organs not used in one locale to other locales. Another aim of these agencies is to provide a supply of donor organs that could match as close as possible potential recipients' tissue-type, size, etc., again so as to increase the probability of a successful transplantation. For instance, highly compatible kidneys are sent to patients already immunised and with high levels of antibodies in the blood, in order to reduce the risk of organ rejection.

The transplantation centres: The transplantation centre is a key node of the network. At such a centre, the acquisition of organs is co-ordinated and transplantations are performed. The country has 5 transplantation centres: Gothenberg, Stockholm, Lund, Uppsala and Malmö. A transplantation centre is a regional hospital attached to a university medical school. The interchange of organs is co-ordinated by the transplantation co-ordinators of the different regions that form an operation network throughout the country and abroad (Scandinavian co-ordinating centres). Each transplantation centre receives organs from hospitals in its region; the transplantation centre at the Sahlgrenska Hospital in Gothenburg operates as national transplantation centre for heart and heart-lung transplantation, thus receiving these organs from the entire country.

A transplantation centre, e.g. for kidneys, has special organisational requirements such as adequate laboratories (for typing, checking of cyclosporine concentration, cytoimmunological analysis, biopsies, etc.), access to an intensive care unit, enough capacity for infection therapy, blood resources, enough equipment to treat all forms of renal insufficiency, anaesthetists, surgeons, etc., working under a 24 hour period. The laboratory is particularly important in the transplantation process, because of the central role prophylactics and therapy plays in avoiding organ rejection.

The donor hospitals: Normally these are the county and municipal hospitals in each region. The care of brain-damaged patients requires some minimum of personnel and technical requirements – satisfied by all the county and municipal hospitals.

The hospital serving the recipient (post-transplantation controls): County hospitals that are in charge of patients with transplants require laboratory resources and adequately trained health-care personnel in order to detect and deal with rejection in its initial phase (Groth 1989: 4591).

Rules and Principles

The different phases of the organ transplantation are organised and regulated according to specific complexes of rules and procedures applied in each phase of the process (see Figure 5). The actors involved have specific roles and functions. The interactions between the actors in the various activity settings is organised and defined by formal and informal rules.

I will illustrate several key rules governing the organisation of the transplantation system, in particular those concerning the selection of organ recipients in the transplantation centre.[33] These rules or criteria for selection of recipients are not enforced by law in Sweden but are general guidelines provided to the transplantation units. One can distinguish three types of criteria:

(1) *Medical technical criteria* (varies with the type of organ, here kidneys): these refer basically to (a) tissue type compatibility, (b) level of antibodies, (c) dialysis time (kidney), (d) general health status, where urgent patients maybe prioritised, (e) body size.

(2) *Administrative criteria*: Waiting time on the list of recipients is the main administrative criteria in the selection of recipients, but also other criteria may play an important part, such as the fair distribution of medical services

(i.e. transplantation surgery) to patients at all the hospitals of the region.

(3) *Psychosocial criteria*: An acceptable level of self-discipline and cooperation on the part of the recipient is considered necessary in the post-transplantation period if eventual rejections are to be avoided. Initial investigations indicate that there are no formalised criteria used in the selection of recipients. In practice, there are various informal rules providing selection criteria: for example, enough psychological stability to go through a long convalescing period; a stable "family" situation, a stable economy and work situation (Hellbom, 1988). Variables such as "quality of life" are very much dependent on this type of criteria.

Key Actors in the Transplantation Process

The physician in care of the potential donor: ICU physicians in care of potential donors are central to the organ procurement since they are responsible for the eventual requests to the family of a deceased regarding organ donation.

The transplantation surgeons and other physicians: The transplantation team consists technically of two groups, the one that extract the organs and the one that perform the operation in the recipient. For extracting a heart, two thorax surgeons, one anesthesiologist, one operation nurse, one anesthesiology nurse and one perfussionist are needed (Transplantationsverksamhet for lever och hjärta; PM: 1988:38).

Transplantation co-ordinator: The main function of a transplantation co-ordinator is to function as a link between the donor hospital and the transplantation centre where the transplantation is performed, as well as maintaining contact with the patients waiting for transplantation. Each centre (Stockholm, Gothenburg, Lund, Malmö, Uppsala) counts with at least two transplantation co-ordinators, specialised in organ procurement and organ recipients. In Scandinavia they are most often specialised nurses and may assist in the organ extraction.

Potential donors: The potential donors as actors are key to the acquisition of organs as long as donation is the accepted form of access to organs for transplantation. Their attitudes are central to the organisation and possibilities of expansion of the system. Their acting capacity is extended beyond death through a donor card or a final will.

Constraints

Characteristic of urgency: The viability of solid organs outside of the donor's body is relatively short (see Table 1). When organs become available,

Figure 4. Transplantation process

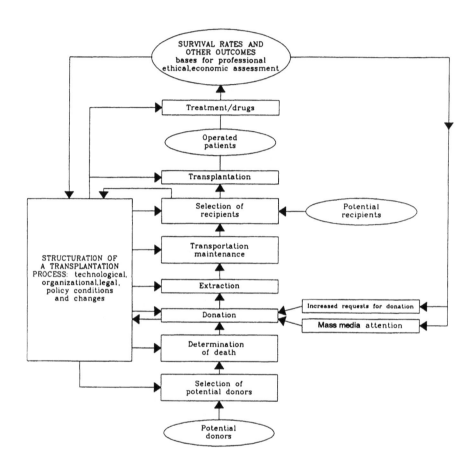

the health-care personnel involved in transplantations has to be available all the time. Since the process can take more than 24 hours, it requires constant availability of surgeons and nurses, laboratory personnel and other professionals to fulfil the requirements.

Transportation constraints: Given that the mortality rate for the recipient increases with each hour that the graft organ to be implanted is outside of the donor's body, rapid transfer is essential. Aeroplane, helicopter and ambulance are the common means used to transport graft organs. The logistics of organ transplantation entail organising the movement of organs, recipients and transplantation teams. Thus, geographical distances, and/or unavailability of adequate means of transportation, may act as constraints on organ exchange between hospitals and regions.

Strategic Resources

Technical resources: drugs, effective technology, etc. Transplantation is basically dependent on immunosuppression therapy that prevents rejection of the graft organ in the body of a patient. In other words, the level of development in immunology is central in making transplantations technically possible.

Human resources: accumulation of expert knowledge, available physicians, technicians and nurses, high levels of organ donation, etc.

Elaborated Flow Model of a Transplantation Process

The flow-chart presented in Figure 6 is the description of a transplantation process in one of the Swedish health care regions. The area covers several counties in the middle regions of the country that are the primary organ harvesting area of the transplantation centre, where transplantations of livers, kidneys and pancreas are currently performed.

Transplantations of minor organs, tissue (for example bone marrow, corneas) and autologic are also performed, but these have other characteristics, due to the use of living donors in the first case and special policies for transplantation of corneas. The flow-chart diagram represents the process of a kidney transplantation. The graft organ comes from a braindead donor. This type of process corresponds also to heart or pancreas donation performed with the aid of a dead donor. Because kidney transplantation is the most common and widely applied, it functions as the base for the organisation of other types of transplants. The main difference with other types of transplants, such as liver or heart

Figure 5. Social rules of a transplantation process

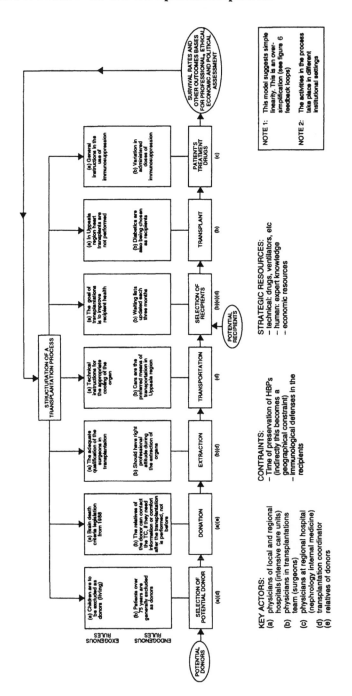

Figure 6. Flow diagram of transplantation processes

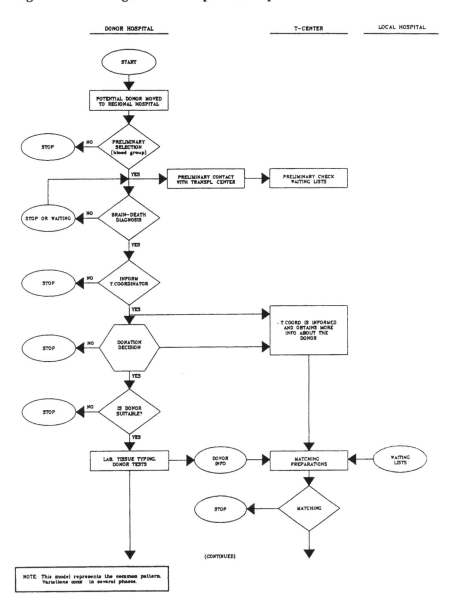

Figure 6a. Flow diagram of transplantation processes (cont.)

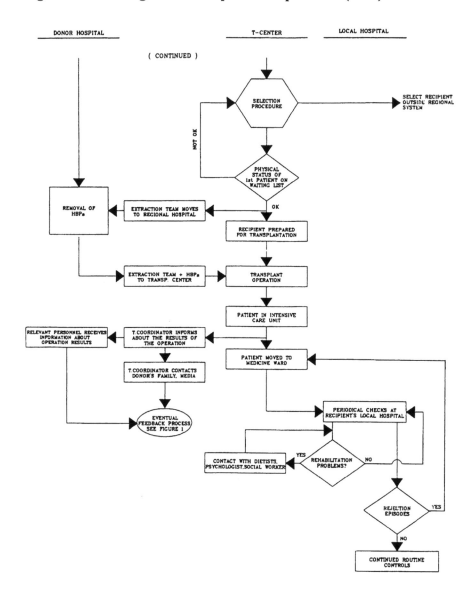

transplantations, is that time marginals for transport and availability of the organs are greater (see Table 1).

Normally, given the consent for donation – and if no specifications are made by the donor while alive or relatives after death – multiple organs are extracted from the donor's body. If more than one organ is taken from the donor, the organs are transported to the transplantation centre of the region where the patient belongs or, in the case of hearts, to Gothenberg, the single transplantation centre which covers the whole country as an operation area for heart transplants. All patients waiting for heart transplantation are connected to this centre. These processes are similar to the one exemplified in Figure 6. There are some sub-processes not included here, such as the process of obtaining organs through international organ exchange networks.

This descriptive model of the organ transplantation process enables the researcher or the practitioner to specify, and to disclose the complex linkages between actors, various settings, phases and types of activity in the overall process, and some of the rules structuring the activities.[34]

Figure 6 provides a detailed flow model representing key activities and choices in the transplantation process – and the action settings and actors involved in these. Figures 4 and 5 present more macro-perspectives. Figure 6, in particular, links institutionalised rules including medical norms and public laws to the transplantation process.

Already in the models presented here, one can identify those phases in the transplantation process that entail a high potential of social tension and conflict, for example around the procurement and selection decisions. Such conflicts can set in motion initiatives to mobilise opinion and support, to bring about new rules and policies through either state or professional regulation, leading to changes in the dynamics of the process (Figure 5).

Notice that at key social or collective decision moments (represented by hexagons in the figures), medical and everyday cultures confront one another – embodied in the participating actors. In the case of organ donation decision-making, the profane perspective of medicine on dead bodies confronts the family (and everyday) perspective that views the dead person as sacred, deserving of special respect and ritual. In the case of recipient selection, dilemmas may arise between decisions based mainly on medical considerations (such as minimising the risk of organ rejection) and consideration of fairness or justice, such as waiting time in a queue. These matters are examined in later chapters.

3 Organ Procurement: Legislation and Praxis

Introduction

The value of human organs and tissue as useful bio-medical materials has increased dramatically in recent years, leading to increased regulation of body part use, in part to prevent abuse, in part to regulate medical access to human tissue and organs. A number of laws and regulations directly concern the citizen's body, alive or dead (i.e. the proper handling of individual persons' bodies and corpses) and several of these regulations are associated with medical procedures such as transplantation, autopsies, criteria for determining death, insemination, castration, research with foetal tissue, the proper handling of corpses, etc. (see Chapter 9).[35] These regulations answer to many interests and rationalities, responding to important social and medical requirements, but they also are expressions of the significant weight and extent of legal control applied to private areas of human existence. Moreover, the regulation of organ access and use has implications far beyond the medical sphere in redefining the boundaries between individual rights, family rights and state rights in dealing with bodies and body parts.

The first two sections of this chapter examine several aspects of laws regulating access to and use of human organs and tissue. The first section identifies patterns of the European (and other OECD countries) legislation relating to organ procurement while the second section examines briefly details of the Swedish law. The final sections discuss the actual patterns of organ donation in a number of countries and the concept of donation.

Transplantation Laws: Comparisons and Patterns

Most countries in Europe have a national transplant law concerning the use of body parts for transplantation. Among the exceptions are Ireland,[36] Holland (until recently);[37] Germany[38] and Switzerland (only some cantons laws and instituted policies that apply to organ procurement and use). For example, in the Netherlands, before the sanctioning of a specific legislation, the Law regulating autopsies was utilised, thus allowing organs to be extracted with the previously expressed consent of the deceased or that of a close relative.

That is, whenever specific actions regarding organ and tissue transfer are not included in a transplantation law, the legality of any actions (e.g. selection of candidates for transplantation, or the legal definition of next-of-kin) is dictated by the general laws applied to medical jurisdiction (e.g. in Sweden, the Health Care Act).

Concerning this, the Council of Europe issued a resolution (78)29 for the harmonisation of the legislation of the member states that was adopted in May 1978 by the Committee of Ministers [of the Council of Europe], recommending policies concerning removal, grafting and transplantation of human substances. The importance of having a legal basis for organ and tissue procurement in Europe is also underscored in other European guidelines such as the 3rd Conference of European Health Ministers (Paris, Nov. 1987), and by the Council of Transplantation. The World Health Organization also issued a series of guiding principles in its Human Organ Transplantation report (1991). These propositions emphasise the importance of the legality regarding organ transplantation and of a harmonisation of European policies. It stresses citizen's consent to such medical procedures and proscribes organ expropriation from the deceased and the commercialisation of organs in the case of living donors.

Necro-Donation

In most European legal provisions concerning the removal of organs and tissue from cadaver donors,[39] the individual donation (whether with presumed consent or not) is regarded as the most legitimate basis for organ and tissue procuring. Legislation in most European countries is based on a policy of presumed consent – organs can be extracted from a deceased unless she expressly objects to this (see Table 4). Some countries (including Sweden between 1988 and 1996) largely rely on voluntary consent. In general, one can distinguish between two types of system, those based on voluntary consent and those based on presumed consent (O'Neill, 1996). These are discussed and illustrated below.

Voluntary Consent Systems: Here we find the Anglo-Saxon countries with their strong normative concepts of individual rights and property rights: England[40] along with Australia, Canada, and the USA. These countries typically launch information and normative campaigns to encourage people to donate, to be "altruistic". This may be accomplished in part by people signing donor cards (Australia, England) or endorsing a driver's licence (as in some states in the USA). While public opinion surveys indicate that most people are positive to organ donation, people exhibit in practice much less readiness. A further problem is that next-of-kin are reluctant to approve a donation if they are uncertain about the wishes of the deceased (see O'Neill, 1996:22). Much more fundamental is the legal uncertainty of "a commitment to donate". Signing a donor card, endorsing a driver's licence, or other means of indicating intention (in contrast to a formal testament with witnesses) are merely expressions of interest, not a legal commitment to donate (O'Neill, 1996:21). O'Neill (1996:21) points out:

> There is no legal contract established and, in the language of the law of contract, making such an indication only represents an 'invitation to treat'. It is extremely unlikely under a system of voluntary consent that any transplant surgeon would remove a deceased individual's organs solely on the basis of a signed donor card or licence. The accepted practice is to seek permission for the donation of organs from next-of-kin.

Presumed Consent Systems: In these systems, individuals are presumed to agree to the donation of their organs unless, at some time during their life, they have indicated otherwise. The burden is on the individual in such a system to "opt-out"of the system if they do not wish to donate their organs.

Typically, countries with presumed consent legislation have a history of a high level of state intervention and/or authoritarian rule. The populations of these countries (Sweden is, in many respects, an exemplary case) have been accustomed to the state intervening in and regulating social life and thus are more disposed to accept legislation that effectively gives the state control over and use of their bodies after death (O'Neill, 1996:24-25). A common practice now in many (but not all) presumed consent countries is the establishment of a registry where those who object to the donation of their organs may have their objection recorded.

According to several European legislations based on presumed consent policies, if the wishes of the deceased are not known, the right to extract organs depends on the wishes or judgement of next-of-kin. Belgium, Italy, Norway, Finland and Sweden give the next-of-kin of a deceased the right to veto organ extraction. Most laws specify that the relatives of the deceased should be informed about their right to object to organ extraction prior to the procedure. However, few countries strictly follow a system where the opinion of the relatives is disregarded. In most countries, the law is more flexible. In any case, doctors are disposed to take into consideration any objection and, in practice, they usually talk with the family of the deceased about organ donation.

In most European laws (except Austria and the Russian Federation), the family acts as "sources of information" about the wishes of the deceased with respect to organ extraction. In France, the transplantation Law allows any person that knew the deceased to witness the deceased's opinion on organ donation, while entering a "substantiated statement" of the particulars.

Table 4. Legal status of donors in selected countries

Donors' legal situation in European countries 1993	
Austria	Presumed consent
Belgium	Presumed consent
Bulgaria	Presumed consent
Cyprus	Presumed consent
Denmark	Presumed consent (strong)
Finland	Presumed consent
France	Presumed consent
Germany	Non-presumed consent (strong) (law approved 1997)
Greece	Presumed consent (but not practised)
Hungary	Presumed consent
Italy	Presumed consent (strong - but not practised)
Japan	Non-presumed consent (strong)
Luxembourg	Presumed consent (but not practised)
Portugal	Presumed consent (but not practised)
Spain	Presumed consent (but not practised)
Sweden	Non-presumed consent (changed to presumed consent 1996)
Switzerland	Presumed/informed consent depending on canton
The Netherlands	Non-presumed consent (strong) (law approved 1996)
UK and Republic of Ireland	Non-presumed consent (strong)

Two forms of the Presumed Consent System can be identified (O'Neill (1996:24): an exclusive or "strong" form in which the family of the deceased is not consulted before organs are taken, and an inclusive or "weak" form which seeks the family's consent to organ donation (although typically this is not a requirement of the presumed consent legislation; Sweden is an exception, see later).

Some argue that a presumed consent system results in higher rates of organ donation. This has been a common argument in Sweden. However, there is great variation in all these systems. Among the countries with the highest rates of donation, Austria has exclusive presumed consent whereas Belgium and Spain have family inclusion. Spain has become an interesting case in part because it has been highly successful in organ procurement at the same time that it has shown a high degree of respect for both potential donors and next-of-kin. It's success depends to a great extent on the way that organ procurement is organised, a key factor being the way that physicians are given incentives to identify potential donors and to persuade families to agree. Procurement in a certain sense is organised and operates as a type of production system (O'Neill, 1996:29-31).

Table 5. Exclusive and inclusive systems

Exclusive systems (relatives not necessarily consulted)	Inclusive systems (relatives necessarily consulted)
Austria, Denmark, Poland, Latvia, Switzerland (partially)	France, Finland, Greece, Italy, Norway, Spain, Sweden (1965-75; 1996-)

In general, a variety of factors affects the supply of organs: the legal restrictions and facilitations, general attitudes among the public to organ transplantation and to the concept of donation; medical contradictions to donation (e.g. drug use, disease); the organisation of procurement (e.g. employment of a procurement co-ordinator); motivation of the procurement surgical team; cooperation of the staff at donor hospitals;[41] opposition from relatives in cases where their views are taken into account; laws regulating procurement or norms that stress respect toward and consideration of the views of the deceased person's next-of-kin; the requirement that hospitals routinely inquire, identify potential organ donors and approach the next-of-kin for consent. In sum, many factors enter in and influence this very complex socio-technical process. The key to understanding the actual procurement levels in any given system is to describe and analyse how the process is organised, how particular actors or groups of agents interact in relation to transplantation activities and the ways in which a matrix of factors influence the course and outcomes of the process.

Living Donation

Medically, living donation has great advantages. Donors and recipients may be genetically related (parent/child, sibling/sibling), although obviously this is not the case between spouses. The transplantation process can be planned and executed under controlled conditions – in this way, the organ (a kidney, a segment of liver) can be transplanted under optimal conditions. On the other hand, organs and organ segments are removed from a healthy, living person. The operation puts a healthy person at risk (no matter how small), and her future life may be jeopardised (one kidney involves more risk than two). The legally unfortunate circumstance of allowing a person to be maimed with the blessing of state laws is tolerated because another person gains in quality of life, if not in life itself. But obviously, there are profound legal as well as ethical issues involved (see Chapter 10) and consequently a general resistance to live donation in several legislations and policy regimes.

The US and most European countries have specific transplant laws dealing with living donation. But few jurisdictions specifically limit permissible transplants from living donors to recipients with whom they have an existing relationship, whether familial (genetic or not) or emotional. One or two countries do have some limited provisions of this kind, although these tend to be linked to other provisions relating to donation by minors. For instance, according to the statutes agreed in the Convention on Human Rights and Biomedicine by the Council of Europe in Oviedo 1997, minors may only donate an organ to a brother or sister and only when the organ/tissue is renewable (Council of Europe, 1997). Most of these norms are followed in the European countries. In all cases, the voluntary consent of the donor is axiomatic, and typically must be expressively given (either in writing or orally in the presence of witnesses).

Similarly, while most legislations prohibit the commercialisation of organ donation, some legal formulations allow for a certain flexibility or permissiveness. For example, the prohibition of trade with human organs and tissue was formulated in Europe as early as 1978 in the form of the Council of Europe's Resolution (78)29 on Harmonisation of Legislations of Members States to Removal, Grafting and Transplantation of Human Substances, adopted by the Committee of Ministers of the Council of Europe on May 1978. While the Article 14 confirms the principle, stating that "a substance must not be offered for any profit". In 1987, at the 3rd Conference of European Health Ministers, the anti-commercial stance was strongly reiterated: "..a human organ must not be offered for profit by any exchange organisation, organ banking centre or any other organisation or individuals whatsoever...". Moreover, to ensure that the donation of an organ is not tainted in any way, it states that the transfer should be totally spontaneous and completely without payment. However, the Article 9 of the Resolution gives the possibility of adhering to the spirit of the law while opening the way to practical solutions:

> ...no substance may be offered for profit. However, loss of earnings and any expenses caused by the removal or preceding examination may be refunded. The donor, or potential donor, must be compensated independently of any possible medical responsibility, for any damage sustained as the result of a removal procedure or preceding examination, under a social security or other insurance scheme.

A Note on Sweden: Shifting Balance of Collective Need and Individual Autonomy

Sweden is a particularly interesting country in that it has shifted over the past 50 years from presumed consent to voluntary consent back again to presumed consent. During this period there has been a substantial development in citizen autonomy and rights.[42] A series of Transplant Acts has been passed, regulating the extraction of organs and tissue from living or deceased human beings for purposes of transplantation.[43] (In Sweden no specific law regulates the allocation of the organs beyond the general regulations for the treatment of patients in health care facilities.)

As in several other technically advanced countries, transplantation surgery developed rapidly in Sweden after the Second World War. The first Act (1958) to regulate organ transplantation came as a codification of prior practices.[44] The "Act on the Use of Tissue and Other Biological Material" regulated the use of corpses for purposes of transplantation and applied the principle of *presumed consent*. Organ or tissue extraction could be performed if the potential donor or the next-of-kin did not explicitly refuse the procedure, or if there were no grounds to believe that they would refuse. Informing the next-of-kin was not, however, mandatory.

In 1975, the second Transplant Act was passed. The rule of presumed consent was left unchanged, but some amendments were introduced. The next-of-kin were to be informed prior to the procedure if possible (if no close relative was available, the organ extraction could be performed). The physician in care of the patient (recipient) could not be the same physician that was in charge of the potential donor. For the extraction of organs for transplantation from living donors, written consent was established as mandatory. If living donors were not legally competent (e.g. minors and mentally handicapped), authorisation of the Board of Health (*Socialstyrelsen*) was required. The use of biological material removed in minor operations was excepted from the jurisdiction of the 1975 Act. In sum, from 1958 until 1987, the *state* (understood as agents such as hospitals, clinics, their representatives, persons of authority) could remove major parts for purposes of transplantation from deceased persons – unless they had explicitly indicated opposition to this.

The issue of presumed consent[45] regarding the extraction of organ and tissue for transplantation was subject to serious debates in connection with a Government bill on Transplantation issues submitted to the Parliament in 1986.[46] Amendments to the 1975 Transplant Act were approved in 1987. In the case of necro-donors, presumption of consent was to be replaced by presumption of non-consent. If no previous written authorisation by the deceased was available, the next-of-kin as representatives of the deceased could authorise the extraction.[47] In constituting the next-of-kin as representative of the will of the deceased, traditional kin rights were to some extent resurrected and a certain legal ambiguity was produced in relation to the individual person's autonomy (see below).[48]

According to the 1975/1987 Act, any legally mentally competent adult was in principle entitled to give tissue, or one of the paired organs, for purposes of transplantation (lungs or eyes are in principle excluded for reasons of serious impairment of the health of the donor). Written consent from the donor and prior information about the procedure was mandatory: no extraction could take place against the donor's will or in her ignorance.[49] Minors or mentally handicapped persons could act as living organ donors (by proxy of their guardians) if this were authorised by the National Board of Health, underscoring the role of the Board of Health in protecting this kind of donor.[50] According to the Act, authorisation was to be granted only if substantial reasons (*synnerliga skäl*) justify it.

No particular restrictions were put on living organ donation as long as the requirement of the written consent from the donor was obtained: no particular familial or other bonds between donor and receiver are specified. However, until recently "living" organ donations have been largely restricted to biologically related donors, or next-of-kin, since organ donation from remote relatives or socially unrelated living donors is viewed as a highly questionable type of action. It is difficult to assess the altruistic motivation in this kind of donation and even so it is ethically difficult to justify the sacrifice. Therefore, medical practice has relied on the familial bonds of next-of-kin[51] or even enduring friendship ties as opposed to donations motivated by any other interest than helping the patient in need of an organ.

Important amendments to the Transplant Act were suggested by the official inquiries in 1989 (SOS:1989:98) and 1992 (SOU 1992:16), and in particular, by the 1995 final Government Proposition (Proposition 1994/1995:148). The inquiry of 1992 (SOU:1992:16) underscored the importance of safeguarding the donor's right to self-determination (including deceased donors), and proposed a unified Act concerning medical and legal actions on bodies, including transplantation, as well as dissection, autopsy, extraction of human biological material for research and pharmaceuticals (from living or deceased), and use of foetuses. Such a "Unified Act" would regulate those medical and legal actions permissible on the human body, whether dead or alive. The intent was to harmonise a complex of laws within a consistent legal frame.

In view of years of preparation, the actual Government Proposition for legislative action and parliamentary consideration (Proposition 1994/95:148) came as a surprise, even to those involved in the 1989 and 1992 inquiries. In contrast to the recommendations of 1989 and 1992 inquiries, the Proposition advocated presumption of consent in the use of body parts for transplantation and other medical purposes, while stressing veto right for relatives. A donor registry would be created. The Act also regulated the use of foetal tissue (previously unregulated by legislation but subject to approval of the ethical committee of the Swedish Medical Society). It restricted the use of dead foetuses requiring informed consent from the woman and special authorisation from the Board of Health. It also rejected the suggestion of a Unified Act, and proposed instead to limit itself to a Transplants Act regarding the transfer of tissue and body parts of living or dead persons for transplantation and other medical purposes.

This final proposition was approved as a law that became effective in July 1996. In general terms, the Act of 1996 follows a policy of harmonisation with other European countries. In this particular Act, the principle of self-determination of the citizens recedes while the principle of collective good occupies a more preferred place. An important ground for a radical change of direction in Swedish policies regarding transplantation appears to have been justified by the generally positive attitude of the Swedish population towards organ donation, and the prospect of increasing the quantity of organs and tissue available for transplantation (Proposition 1994/95:148).

Donation in Practice: Beyond the Legislation

As pointed out above, there is considerable variation in the transplantation laws from country to country, for example, with respect to presumed or non-presumed consent. Consent laws and policies also may vary over time, as we have seen in the case of Sweden. The wide variation in legal regulation – between presumed consent and non-presumed consent – is *not* correlated strongly with levels of donation. For example we find presumed consent in countries such as Italy (requiring approval from the family) with very low donation rates; the UK with non-presumed consent has a relatively high donation rate (see Figure 7). Belgium and France – also with presumed consent policies – have low donation rates. The country with by far the highest donation rate, Spain, has presumed consent and requires consultation with next-of-kin.

If legislation is not decisive, then what are the key factors affecting donation? Legislation may have more to do with political culture and religious ideas than with the necessity of organ procurement or rational arguments about such needs. Besides legal regulations, other factors affecting organ donation rates are: a percentage of braindead are medically unsuitable as donors; failure to detect potential donors, reluctance to ask relatives about organ donation; and the relatives refusal of to allow organ extraction (Miranda and Matesanz, 1996); technical factors (problems of storage and transportation, etc.); the organisation of procurement. Several social and legal factors have contributed to reducing the quantity of organs available in later years. For example, the introduction of laws making the use of security belts in driving mandatory and similar measures have reduced the severity and number of traffic accidents, bringing about a reduction of potential donors. In addition, the techniques to treat such cases have improved (Briggs et al., 1997).

Figure 7. Donation patterns in selected countries and regions

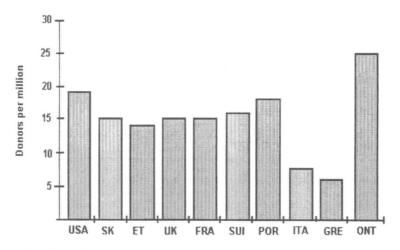

SK: Scandiatransplant: Denmark, Finland, Norway, Sweden.
ET: Eurotransplant: Austria, Belgium, Germany, The Netherlands.
UKTSSA: United Kingdom Transplant Support Service Authority: United Kingdom and Republic of Ireland.
ONT: Spain; FRA: France; ITA: Italy; SUI: Switzerland; GRE: Greece.

Source: ONT, Spain 1994 Donation Rates.

Non-technical factors – professional doubts about organ transplantation or brain death, unwillingness to disturb grieving relatives, lack of time or problems to identify potential donors and organisational problems – together with family refusals, appear to be equally as important as legislative measures of non-presumed consent in constraining organ procurement. In any case, there is considerable variations in donation patterns between countries (see Figure 7 and also Table 2 in Chapter 2) – but also between regions and local transplantation centres, within any region or country.

Characteristics of Organ Donors

There is a wide variation in the characteristic of organ donors, since the causes and rates of death are strongly dependent on the particular social and cultural characteristics of each country or even region.

Brain death: The potential donor pool has been estimated as possibly 50 donors per million population/year, but the actual rates of necrodonation for many countries are significantly lower. For example, in Scandinavia in 1996 the total number of donors was 14.6 donors per million population (Madsen et al., 1997). In spite of most European legislations establishing presumed consent for the extraction of cadaveric organs for transplantation, organ donation rates depend on many other factors, as pointed out earlier.

Accidents/disease: Some years ago most potential braindead donors were typically victims of accident-caused trauma, sudden acute illness, violence, or self inflicted injury (JAMA,1985; Martyn et al., 1988; Steuer and Bell, 1989, Yanaga et al., 1989). For example, in 1991 nearly 60% of the brain death donors in Spain were cerebrovascular victims (Transplant, 1991/1992). In the USA, motor vehicle accidents as a cause of death of organ donors decreased from 34% to 22% between 1988 and 1993, while cerebrovascular deaths increased from 28% to 37% during the same time period. In the Scandinavian countries, in 1996, patients suffering spontaneous cerebral haemorrhage made up 73% of the total of donors while 15% were the result of accidents (Madsen et al., 1997). In general, in many countries today more cases of brain death result from spontaneous cerebral haemorrhage or stroke, than from head traumas. However, accidents still make up a relatively high proportion of the organ sources in the 1990s, as much as 49% in France, 41% in Eurotransplant, 30% in the UK, 43% in Switzerland, and 40% in Spain (Miranda and Matesanz, 1996).

Age: The age pattern of organ sources has also shifted, from quite young organ donors some years ago to older donors in latter years. For example, in Spain since 1989 the number of organ donors between 15-29 years has decreased from 45 to 25%, while more than 20% are older than 60 years (Miranda and Matesanz, 1996). In the Scandinavian region, in 1996, 41% of the donors were between 40 and 59 years old whereas 17% were 60 years old or more (Scandiatransplant, 1997). The increased age of organ donors has been explained by several factors such as a decrease in traffic accidents (Gäbel et al., 1990) and increased use of older graft organs. In the US, cadaveric donors over 50 years old increased from 12% in 1988 to 24% in 1995, while donors in the 18-34 age decreased from 41% of donors in 1988 to 29% of donors in 1995 (UNOS Annual Report, 1996).

Gender: Significantly more men than women become cadaveric organ sources. These figures do not mean that men are more willing to donate but that in general men, more often than women, become organ donors through accidents or illness. For example, in Spain 1991, 67% of the donors were male (Transplant, 1991/1992), and in Australia/New Zealand 61% of the donors (1993-1996) were male (ANZOD, 1997). One explanatory factor is the lower mortality of females in traffic accidents (Beirness, 1989; Bailey, 1989 Öström and Eriksson, 1989).[52] In the US in 1995, males represented 60% of all cadaveric donors (but only 43% of living donors) (UNOS Annual Report, 1996). A study performed in order to map the number of potential organ donors in Sweden, from 1989 to 1991, showed that men were somehow overrepresented in necrodonation. Of 299 individuals that became organ donors, 177 were men (59%) and 122 were women (41%). It must be stressed, however, that men significantly outnumber women among patients dying under ventilator treatment (62% versus 38% (Gäbel and Edström, 1992)).

Attitudes Towards Organ Donation

Surveys in Europe, Australia and North America consistently find positive attitudes to cadaveric donation. For example, a 1993 Gallup survey on public attitudes to organ donation in the US showed a general support (85%) for the concept of cadaveric organ donation while 15% were undecided or negative about it (Gallup, 1993). A similar study for Boston (commissioned by the New England Organ Bank, USA in 1993) showed that 72% of respondents wanted to donate their organs after death. The Organ Donation Attitudes Research in Australia (ACCORD, 1995) indicated that 90% of the Australian population in principle support organ donation (26% of the population had decided to become donors, 23% "probably" intended to become donors, 33% were undecided while 18% refused to donate). In Sweden the pattern of support for organ donation shows that 70% of the population is positive to organ donation (Proposition 1994/95:148).

Standard background variables such as age, gender and education relate to attitudes toward organ donation, as indicated in Table 6. Common attitudes associated with doubts about or opposition to donation are: disbelief in brain death, insistence on maintaining bodily integrity, fear that doctors may not try as hard to save the patient if she is a donor, worry that the donation process might upset the family, belief that one is too old for organ donation, fear of experiencing pain, religious barriers (ACCORD, 1995; Persjin et al., 1997; Sanner, 1991; Matesanz and Miranda, 1996). Another common attitude found in several studies is that willingness to receive organs is greater than to donate them (Gäbel and Lindskoug, 1989; SOU:1989:99; Persjin et al., 1997). According to Spanish and French studies, common reasons for families to refuse donation are the belief that the deceased was opposed to donation, family opposition regardless of the attitude of the deceased, unclarity concerning brain death, and concerns about body integrity (Gomez and Santiago, 1995; Fernandez Lucas et al., 1996).

Table 6. Attitudes towards organ donation

	Attitudes toward organ donation
General attitude	Positive in countries where survey results available*
Readiness to donate	Generally positive but the percentage expressing readiness to donate is significantly lower than those expressing approval of organ donation
Age	Young people are more positive than older people
Gender	Minimal difference between women and men in rates of approval and disapproval. Women however exhibit more undecidability than men
Education	The higher the level of education the greater the level of approval

* Surveys: UNOS, 1996; ANZOD, 1996; Gallup, 1993; Gäbel et al., 1989, 1991; Sanner, 1991; Roels et al., 1997.

Living Donation

Many transplantations of kidneys, but also segments of liver and parts of the bowels, pancreas and lung are performed using organs from living donors (Blohmé et al., 1992), (Francis et al., 1992), (Evans, 1992), (Faltin et al., 1992).

The main reason for relying on living donors is the scarcity of cadaveric organs to cover the organ demand, and the excellent transplantation results with organs from genetically related donors. A third reason for using living donors is that some countries lack sufficient economic and sociotechnical resources to manage a sufficiently large cadaveric pool, and transplantations performed with living donors do not require such a complex sociotechnical infrastructure. Transplantation models based primarily on cadaveric donation are the most frequent patterns in Europe and in the Americas. However, the number of living donors is substantial in a number of countries (see Table 7).

Table 7. Living and necrodonation

	Living donation	**Cadaveric donation**
Greece (1985-1990)[53]	58%	42%
Norway (1988-1992)[54]	43%	57%
Sweden (1994-1995)[55]	32%	68%
Italy (Central/Southern)[56]	32%	68%
Denmark (1991-1994)[57]	26%	74%
USA	21%	79%
Finland (1991-1994)[58]	5%	95%
Hungary (1982-1990)[59]	5%	95%
Switzerland (1987-1990)[60]	3%	97%
Portugal (1991)[61]	0%	100%

This Table indicates the ratio of necrodonation and living donation for several European countries and the US.[62]

Living Donation and Gender

Even if women are significantly underrepresented as cadaveric donors, there are strong indications that women are substantially overrepresented as living donors in a number of countries (see Table 8). Moreover, a large percentage of living donation is from women to men, especially mothers to their children (O'Neill, 1996). The tables quantify what transplantation surgeons have indicated in interviews, namely that women appear to donate more while alive than men. And women also appear to receive less (see Chapter 4).

Table 8. Living donation by gender in selected countries

	Totals	Women	Men
Eighth Report (1967-1969)[63]	n.a.	56%	44%
Norway (1988-1992)[64]	389	60%	40%
Hannover (1973-1989)[65]	83	64%	36%
Gothenburg (1981-1989)[66]	276	59%	41%
Glasgow (1969)[67]	138	57%	43%
Greece (1968-1989)[68]	n.a.	63%	37%
Iran (1984-1989)[69]	185	57%	43%
Minnesota * (pancreas) (1966-1990)[70]	36	65%	35%
Minnesota ** (pancreas) (1966-1990)[71]	76	67%	33%
Melbourne[72]	n.a.	77%	23%
Chicago (liver) (1990)[73]	16	63%	37%
Chicago (liver) (1989-1991)[74] **	n.a.	65%	35%

Source: see respective notes.

Organ Donation as Giving, Exchanging and Extracting

Numerous empirical studies report variation in readiness to donate and in donation patterns, for example:

- that altruism is stronger in closed groups, such as the family and least for foreigners (Vicusi et al., 1988); that while 70% of Americans are generally willing to donate, this willingness decreases when they must act concretely such as signing a donor card and making concrete commitments (Lee and Kissner, 1986).
- that requests for donation in practice put stress on the family of the deceased (Martyn et al.,1988), since even in countries where there is no legal requirement to consult next-of-kin, they are consulted and often determine the final result. Frequently encountered issues among relatives that have been approached and refused to donate are: difficulties understanding the concept of brain death, lack of information about the donor's wishes, concerns about the integrity of the corpse, among other things (Santiago and Gomez, 1997).

- that cultural differences affect patterns of donation (Locke and Honde, 1990). Several studies found a greater reluctance to donate organs among minorities than among other groups. This relates to mistrust of authorities, mistrust of brain death criteria, concerns regarding the mutilation of the corpse of the relative, and more overt expressions of grief [that made communication (organ request) difficult]. Such patterns have been pointed out for black Americans in particular (Davidson and Devney, 1991; Callender et al., 1982) and among non-whites in general in the US (Gallup, 1993); for Hispanics families in Puerto Rico (Fernandez et al., 1991); and for immigrants/ foreigners in Sweden (less prone to donate than born Swedes) (Gäbel et al., 1989). A problem with this type of explanation is the tendency to attribute low donation rates to social traits of the minorities themselves, overlooking organisational and interactive factors (e.g. social, ethnic or behavioural commonalities or differences between procurement teams and relatives of deceased).

There have been several attempts to explain donation behaviour. Underlying these models are conceptions of "altruism".[75] The act of giving in donation has been analysed by Simmons et al. (1977). Their work does not devote itself to conceptualising altruism but their model points at a series of factors predisposing living donation: structural factors (age, sex similarity, position in the family etc.), intervening emotions (emotional closeness, etc.), and situational variables (request actually made or not). As motivation for donation of necroorgans two reason were given: altruism and feelings of continuation of life through the giving of the organ.

The role of altruism in social behaviour has been discussed by a number of social scientists, even in relation to blood and organs (among others Arrow (1981), Titmuss (1971), Walzer (1983), Wolfe (1989)). Titmuss (1971), for example, argued that the commercialised blood markets were inferior to systems of voluntary donors because the latter were more regular, predictable and administratively more efficient and, above all, less likely to distribute contaminated blood. They fostered social integration, contributing to the sense of belonging and participation among members of a community, thus encouraging further altruism. Arrow's (1981) position (in agreement with Titmuss) is that in an economic transaction, the quality of an uncertain good (i.e. blood) cannot be guaranteed if the buyer does not have sufficient knowledge about the good (i.e. information control): therefore, truthfulness is essential in avoiding risk to recipients, for example in the case of blood. Nevertheless, he also pointed out that the market increased the freedom of choice without taking away the right to give freely and that a system of voluntary donation could also prove inefficient if potential donors hesitated to donate, believing that their blood was of poor quality.

In explaining the individual motivation to donate, Titmuss emphasises the desire to benefit others and feelings of social obligation as well as a response to psychological pressures. Arrow puts the stress on the role of self-interest behind altruistic actions. He explains such self-interest in terms of three factors: (1) the pleasure anybody feels when seeing that somebody else's satisfaction increases, (2) the pleasure of being himself/herself the giver, and (3) the calculation that in the short or the long run he/she will benefit by the altruistic action (Arrow, 1981). Hansson (1992) points out that the first explanation in Arrow's model is not applicable to donation to *unknown* recipients; and that the third one can be explained by Titmuss's social obligation.

Common to these analyses about altruism, voluntariness, and markets in relation to organ tissue donation is a highly decontextualised model of human action, minimising the normative bases and different forms of "giving".

Different Forms of Donation

The act of giving may imply an agreed reciprocity, an implicit reciprocity or no reciprocity at all. The first case can in principle be understood as a *market exchange*, the second as a *social exchange* (gift relationship) and the third as a *sacrificial* one.[76]

In the *market exchange*, the logic of calculation in the transactions is focused on the exchange of objects or services between "independent" transactors, the transaction is temporary, contractual and regulated by market rules. A situation of pure market exchange in transplantation would be the sale of organs and tissue. This type of transaction involving payment to living donors is banned in most legislation and is not to be understood as donation.[77]

The *social exchange* type entails a symbolic action and emphasises the establishment and maintenance of social relationships (Burns et al, 1985). In this exchange the axis of the transaction lies in the relationship itself, consequently the commodity given cannot be separated from the relationship, in a sense merging with goods and services. In contrast to market transactions, the goods and services exchanged are defined as so inherent to the relationship that they become part of it (e.g. in parenthood the "gift" of food to the young is inherent to the role as parent). The basic traits of gift relations entail the inalienability of the gift as part of the giver, the obligation to repay the gift, and the generation and regeneration of the relationship as its central and symbolic aspect (Mauss, 1954:78). The concept of gift as a form of exchange is the reaffirmation of a social relationship (or a system of social relations) marked by continuity (obligation to repay in one or other way). Living related organ donation (genetically related = next-of-kin), entails a social exchange, or what is also referred to as "gift exchange".[78]

Living donation, and necrodonation (giving consent to a *future* organ extraction (i.e. after death)) are different actions embodying different norms and social meanings. In *living donation* the distance between attitude, intention and its realisation is short. In necrodonation the distance is in a certain sense infinite.[79] Giving an organ to a close friend or a child is often associated with strong emotions, even with intense religious overtones (Simmons et al., 1977). Additionally, as some living donors report, their decision to give an organ to a relative was less the result of moral reflections or calculations, and more a spontaneous feeling of doing what was evidently right (Simmon et al., 1977). This sense of "obviousness or rightness" tended to follow the family or kinship structure, and patterns of obligations and rights.

The family structure defines roles such as "mother", "father", "sister" etc., where each role connotes particular positional rules, normatively defined as rights and duties. Parents, in particular mothers, reported the donation as self-evident and unambiguous. According to Simmons et al. (1979), the most unproblematic were: from mother to daughter/son; followed by father to daughter/son; followed by wife to husband; husband to wife; unmarried sister to brother; and so on. For example, the living donation from a child to her/his parent was considered problematic in the sense of "unnatural" (for both the parents herself/himself and the health care personnel involved).

In *necrodonation,* as the written or verbal promise of donation of organs in the future, after death, has been connected to values such as "civil responsibility" or "community concerns" (Gäbel and Kelleberg, 1992); to utilitarian considerations about the practicality of recycling the bodies of the dead (Tänsjö, 1990) or to rational calculations about one's future needs (i.e. one might need an organ in the future) (SOU:1989:98). Typical of philosophical discourses about necrodonation is its general and decontextualised character both in its principalist, rational or utilitarian variants (abounding in concepts such as "citizenship", "responsibility", "rationality" or "motherland"), applicable to anybody and to nobody. While living donation patterns follow the pattern of the existing social roles, necrodonation follows abstract principles or non-empirically sustainable calculations.

In *sacrificial giving*, the items or services given are supposed to be irrespective of the act of giving. The role of the receiver as eventual retributor can be secondary (giving to the poor) or more central as part of the role relationship (a soldier dying for his king). For the giver, however, the expectancy of reciprocity is non-existent or negligible. As the motive/ reward of the action is in the act itself, the sacrificial giving can be analysed as the reinforcement of a sense of generalised (social) identity of the giver, as a socio-psychological affirmation as giver (active role) enacting the socio-culturally meaningful values of his reference group. Hansson (1992) has argued that this would not explain actions of giving outside of the sphere of the reference group, but at least in principle the reference group of an individual can became large enough to include all other individuals, as for example in humanitarian or religious views, or even large enough to include, for example, animals. Necrodonation can be understood as sacrificial giving in its more weak variant, almost a sense of civil duty.[80]

Why Donation is Not Simply Donation?

There is a fundamental problem using the term "donation", suggesting "voluntary giving" – with a strong sense of intentionality – to refer to all of the many forms of organ procurement. One should at least make distinctions such as the following:

(1) a person explicitly, consciously, chooses to donate her organs. Surely, those who register themselves, sign a card, communicate to relatives, or take other explicit action, can be considered "donors" in a genuine sense.

(2) proxy donation (see note 14) entails the conscious choice of next-of-kin to donate necro-organs of deceased relatives.

(3) necrodonations in countries with presumed consent may not involve donation in any strict sense of the concept, if the sources of organs have not reflected on the matter or made a decision to donate. The aspect of intentionality is simply missing.

There are certainly borderline cases: people who are aware of a transplant law or policy maintaining presumed consent but passively accept the policy, for one or another reason: too much trouble to register refusal; uncertainty about feelings on the matter; indecidability; genuine indifference. Such passive acceptance cannot be called "donation" and should not be honoured with the designation of "altruism". In general, donation is socially and psychologically a highly ambiguous concept.

4 Recipient Selection: Regulation and Patterns

Introduction

Selection refers to the process whereby patients in need of an organ are selected as recipients (see Chapter 2). Here we are interested in how this process is organised, the norms and rules guiding and regulating selection, and the dilemmas and predicaments that arise in connection with recipient selection and organ allocation. Typically, there is not one but multiple decisions and selection mechanisms in referral networks and eventually in the allocation procedures at the centres where organs are made available.

The criteria for allocating organs for transplantation vary widely, since they differ not only for the different types of organ (one of the main differences regarding the allocation of large organs is between renal and non-renal organs) but also between transplant programs by country, region and even medical centre. Roughly, the process can initially be described as follows:

(1) Patients are identified and proposed by their physicians or hospital teams. Principally, the question of the allocation rules for organs becomes actual once a patient is admitted on a waiting list for receipt of an organ.

(2) But admittance (the initial selection) entails already the application of particular rules (applying medical and non-medical criteria of selection). Patients are proposed who satisfy specific medical criteria such as "no confounding ailments" or "likelihood that the patient will survive the operation" (O'Neill, 1996:51). Non-medical criteria such as age and life-style (for example, no drug or alcohol dependency, capacity to follow a strict drug regime, etc.) are taken into account, usually in an informal way. Even personal and family conditions – such as degree of support – may be initial selection factors in gaining a place in a transplant program (O'Neill, 1996:51).

(3) Once on a waiting list, patients' selection [prioritisation] will depend on the particular rules or procedures utilised in making selection or allocating organs. As discussed below, the procedures and the organisation of the organ procurement and allocation network vary considerably. The distribution of solid organs to those on transplant waiting lists is based on a combination of measures of compatibility or match between donated organs and particular patients, the medical needs of the patient (including the urgency of obtaining a transplant and the degree of immunity reactivities),

and various non-medical factors such as fairness or distributive justice, and social and psychological characteristics of the patient.

Three of the most common criteria used in selection of organ recipients are medical criteria: (1) compatibility of blood types; (2) degree of match of tissue types, which is to a greater or lesser extent inversely related to strong immunological response of the recipient; (3) the degree of immunological hyper-sensitivity (that is, patients with highly reactive antibodies that dispose them to reject transplants).

Blood type compatibility is an absolute requirement, and is rigorously applied in all allocation systems. The application of this rule results, however, in problems of equity: A source of "natural inequality" and inequalities in organ distribution arise because of the incompatibilities of blood types. Persons with type O blood are universal donors, but may receive only from O. Type AB is a universal recipient. A, B, and AB can be crossed.[81]

Table 9. Blood type compatibility

Recipient	Possible Donors
AB	AB, A, B, O
A	A,O
B	B,O
O	O

Another general consideration is the degree of matching of tissue types (that is human leukocyte antigen measures HLA) between donor organ or tissue and recipient.[82] "Tissue matching", "antigen matching", and HLA matching refer to comparison of genetically controlled markers on white blood cells (Dennis, 1991:21). Tissue type compatibility is more flexible that that of blood type – in part because there is some disagreement among specialists about the exact significance of such compatibility. Many judge that the chance of success of a transplant are greater when there is a high degree of compatibility between leukocyte antigens (HLA) of the organ and those of the recipient (an antigen is any substance that can induce a specific immune response), thus decreasing the likelihood of strong immunological response.[83] Some organ allocation systems give major weight in their selection and allocation judgements to the degree of matching (see below). Others give less weight, particularly in view of the availability of powerful immuno-suppressants used today to prevent rejection. Transplant physicians and histocompatibility experts generally agree that a recipient closely matched with a donor enhances long-term graft survival (Dennis, 1991:9). There is less consensus about whether 3 and 4 HLA matched recipients do significantly better than 1 and 2 HLA matched recipients, in part because of the successful use of cyclosporine to limit host rejection of poorly matched kidneys.

The survival of grafts is not only a matter of matching. Recipient reactivity is also of great significance. People vary in their response to a bee sting, or other allergens. Similarly, there are significant differences in the tendency of individuals to mount an aggressive immune response against a graft. In patients with high levels of antibodies – following pregnancy, blood transfusion, or reject of a graft – the outlook for a successful renal graft is poor.

There exists a test, antibody screening, which reveals the extent to which a patient has antibody reactions to other Human Leukocyte Antigens (Punch, 1998). It utilises a sample of different HLAs from a population. It is conducted by mixing a very small amount of the patient's serum with an equal amount of cells from, for instance, *60 different individuals* in a series of tests. In this way, one can determine how many different HLA antibodies a patient has in their blood. This enables one to avoid those antigens when selecting an appropriate donor. If the patient does not have any HLA antibody, the test result will be negative.

The procedure also identifies how much HLA antibody the patient has. For example, if the patient reacts with 54 of the 60 cells, then the patient is said to have 90% antibody, for that particular serum date. This percent antibody is called the Percent Reactive Antibody (PRA). Thus, the antibody screening provides important pieces of information about the patient's serum: (1) the PRA (how much antibody is present); (2) the Specificity (the specific HLA antibody). Since HLA antibody goes up and down, antibody screening is performed regularly, for instance every month.

Hyperimmunised patients are a class that are given special consideration in most systems, since they are highly disposed to reject transplants. The PRA (for instance PRA>80%) is the common operationalisation of hyperimmunisation.

Beyond these basic medical criteria, other factors are introduced such as, distance between the organ source and the hospital of the recipient, waiting time, and balance or fairness between organs provided or donated and organs received in the exchange in a network. Consideration is taken of how long a patient has been waiting (on a waiting list). In many systems this is a consideration and is seen as a matter of equity or fairness. However, even other non-medical factors may enter in. For example, a patient may be given priority because she comes from a hospital or region that regularly provides organs, but has not received many; or it's been a long time since a recipient has been selected from the particular hospital or region.

Some allocation systems explicitly take into account a wide range of factors (Eurotransplant and The United Network for Organ Sharing in the USA), others limit the factors explicitly taken into account in allocation

(Scandiatransplant or France Transplant), as outlined below. Consideration may even be taken of an individual's character and potential social support, since these are believed to play a role in a recipient's close adherence to the post-transplant treatment regime. Correspondingly, there is considerable scepticism and reluctance to transplant to alcoholics or drug addicts (although such views are typically not formalised in particular policies or regulations), not only because their general ill-health is likely to decrease the probability of a successful transplant but because they may be seen as undeserving in any comparison with other potential recipients (and the legitimacy of the allocation system and readiness of people to donate to it depends on beliefs in its fairness and effectiveness in the use of organs).

In sum, general sets of criteria used in selection processes can be distinguished: (1) medical criteria; (2) practical matters of transport, storage and logistics generally; (3) social, psychological, and bio-social criteria; (4) normative (e.g. matters of fairness or justice) (these are analytic distinctions; in practice, they overlap).

Organisation of Organ Allocation

While the medical criteria for allocation are relatively straightforward and universal, their weightings may differ substantially (see below) and the social organisation in which they are applied may vary considerably. Eurotransplant with five European countries (Austria, Belgium, Luxembourg, the Netherlands, and Germany) has a highly centralised organ exchange and allocation organisation. Spain has a highly decentralised system, where most organs are procured locally and transplanted locally. The USA's United Network for Organ Sharing (UNOS) is also mixed, but with considerable centralisation. The Scandinavian countries, who belong to and participate in Scandiatransplant, have a mixed system, but relatively less centralised.

Some OTSs put a great emphasis on an algorithm (possibly based on a complex point system). Others stress flexibility and organic judgement, trying to weigh, balance, etc. more or less on a case-to-case basis. Some OTSs have centralised lists and allocation, others relatively local or decentralised lists. Some combine the two, e.g. France Transplant (the Etablissement Français des Greffes) where one kidney is kept locally and one given to the central allocating office. [84]

Such arrangements are not however ad hoc. They are patterned with a social logic or rationality characteristic of any socially constructed arrangement (see Chapter 5). In the following discussion, I shall briefly describe a highly centralised (typically also formalised) and decentralised system (usually non-formalised, although this may vary).

Large-Scale Centralised Systems

Eurotransplant[85] (Austria, Belgium, Germany, Luxembourg, and the Netherlands) is a good example of a centralised system operating with clearly specified rules for allocating organs to patients on a waiting list. Here we concentrate on kidneys. These are distributed among potential recipients according to a rule complex (in the form of a computer algorithm) applied to a waiting list. Inclusion on the waiting list is the responsibility of each transplantation centre.

A transplantation centre in any of the five countries proposes a transplantable patient to Eurotransplant, providing key data on the patient:

- blood type (allowing for judgement about blood type compatibility)[86]
- HLA data (allowing for judgement concerning tissue type compatibility)
- mismatch probability (that is, probability that a patient with a particular profile is likely to find a match from a population of donors)[87]
- distance/time to transport organ to patient[88]
- effective waiting time[89]
- national import/export balance[90]

The current allocation system is designed to catch all these factors in a total sum for each patient. Each factor is assigned a value on a scale of 1-100. For instance, if tissue type is fully matched to the donor, the highest possible number of points, 100, is scored for this variable. On the other hand, with no match, the patient receives zero points.[91] Then each factor score is weighted from 1 to 4. The highest weight (4) is given to matching, followed by low distance between donor and transplant unit (2.6). Waiting time and national import/export balance are each weighted by a factor of 2. Mismatch probability is weighted by 1. The total point count for each patient is determined by adding up all the scores of the five factors. The higher the total score, the more favourable the assessment. The patient(s) with the highest number of points has first access to an available kidney.

There are various *default rules* which bypass the system above. Simultaneous transplantation of a kidney and any non-renal organ (e.g. pancreas, liver, heart, or lung) has priority over all categories of a kidney-only transplant patient. These cases also take precedence over patients selected according to the "Highly Immunised Patients" program[92] and/or patients selected by the "Acceptable Mismatch" program. All remaining potential recipients are sorted according to their point score, as outlined above. Special points may be awarded for particular types of cases, thus shifting the ranking of patients on the waiting list. If a kidney transplant candidate has the urgency code "High Urgency", the transplant candidate may receive 300 extra points, assigned upon approval by the medical staff of Eurotransplant.[93] In case of a paediatric transplant candidate (< 16 years old) placed on a waiting list, *a bonus waiting time* is assigned, adding to the effective waiting time of the candidate. For instance, candidates younger than 6 years old at the time of listing are assigned a bonus of 1095 days (and the bonus remains until the candidate becomes 16 years old). Transplant candidates between 6 and 11 years of age are assigned a bonus of 365 days. At 11 years of age, the bonus is increased to 730 days.

Decentralised or Substantially Decentralised Systems

Spain is characterised by a decentralised system but with broad agreement on medical and ethical criteria of allocation. There are 33 Kidney transplant centres, six of which are paediatric centres. Each has its own waiting list. Each transplant team has the opportunity to graft all organs generated in the hospital where it is based and in all hospitals from which it receives renal patients. Allocation criteria are strictly decided by the transplant team (together with the regional and national programs for prioritisation of children and hyperimmunised patients). The most suitable match of organ donated and recipient is sought, a principle applied to a greater or lesser extent in all sub-systems. And there is to be no unfair consideration of a geographical nature, or with respect to race, sex, religion, or age.

The central office of the Spanish National Organisation of Transplants (ONT) is responsible for the kidney allocation for hyperimmunised patients. The office maintains the hyperimmunised waiting list, distributes serum samples to all tissue typing laboratories each 3-4 months, and is responsible for the direct observation of the offer and exchange rules accepted previously by the kidney transplant teams (Matesanz and Miranda, 1996).

There are two national regimes for hyperimmunised patients:
- Plan 1: allocation based on HLA compatibility
- Plan 2: allocation based on (-) cross-match with stored serum.

In Spain the allocation of kidneys for transplantation is "...strictly decided by the transplant team with regional programs" (Matesanz and Miranda, 1996:177). However, all Spanish transplant centres participate in regional programs of kidney exchange with respect to the prioritisation of children and hyperimmunised patients. This means that, for these particular cases, the allocation becomes regionally/nationally centralised. The national ONT also collaborates in the allocation of organs when there are no adequate local recipients. Livers and hearts are also allocated locally except for O-urgency patients, regarded as national priority.[94]Whenever a tissue typing laboratory obtains a sample from a kidney that could be grafted into a patient included in the hyperimmunised waiting list, the organ must go to that patient. The ONT central office   arranges the transfer if necessary. The office also maintains data about specifically difficult kidneys (e.g. blood group AB), or paediatric donors under 20 Kg, etc. In case a transplantation centre has no suitable local recipient, the central office of ONT collaborates in searching for an adequate recipient within the rest of the transplant lists.

The ONT in Spain (1996:165) advocates a decentralised system, arguing that organ priority should be given to the area procuring organs. This makes for "geographical fairness" in organ sharing, in the sense that the local transplant centre serves the interests of its community, ensuring legitimacy and effective commitment of members of the community to continue donating organs that are transplanted to their neighbours. This is for them an obvious moral imperative.

However, it is generally recognised that there is a need to also share organs across the borders of communities and regions, not only to avoid wastage (organs unused because of lack of a suitable recipient) but to assure the most suitable match of organ procured and recipient is the objective (the larger the pools of procured organs and potential recipients, the greater the likelihood of a good match). But also to avoid privileges and a sense of unfairness.

Sweden: Decentralisation also characterises Sweden, where each centre is free to determine its own selection criteria. In Sweden (and in general, in Scandinavia), the transplantation centres mainly use the same criteria of selection: blood and tissue compatibility, waiting time, level of immunisation, personal and social situation. But the centres weigh these factors differently. Matching is given more weigh in one centre and less in another, and similarly for waiting time and other considerations (such variation is also found in international comparisons).

Mixed Allocation Systems

Scandiatransplant serves the Scandinavian region (Denmark, Finland, Norway and Sweden), maintaining waiting lists of all the transplant centres of the Scandinavian countries (see Table 2 in Chapter 2). While it co-ordinates the allocation of an important part of the available kidneys (somewhat less than 20% in the past ten years as compared to around 40% the previous 10 years), it does not exercise the degree of organ allocation control that characterises Eurotransplant. Its allocation rules stress donor/organ compatibility. Compulsory exchange with respect to the Scandiatransplant waiting list are as follows (Madsen et al., 1997):

1. Candidates who are HLA-A, -B, -DR compatible with the organ donor, that is zero mismatch.

2. Potential recipients (PRA > 80%) who have HLA-A, -B compatibility with the donor (that is, less compatibility than in Principle 1) and who are hyperimmunised (PRA > 80%).

3. Blood group O and B kidneys should only be used for blood type O and blood group B recipients respectively.

Scandiatransplant has also reciprocity rules: a kidney received by one centre from another must be paid back within a 6 month period with a kidney of the same type. There is no particular criteria regarding the prioritisation of children who are encouraged to receive a living related organ donation. Whenever a Nordic organ cannot be used within the Scandiatransplant area, it is offered to other transplantation allocation organisations, mostly Eurotransplant and United Kingdom Transplant (Madsen et al., 1997: 3987).

The United Network for Organ Sharing (UNOS) in the US is a nationally organised organ (kidney) allocation system. Transplant candidates are registered at their respective transplantation centres but may also be on other regional and national waiting lists. The national waiting list is maintained by the United Network for Organ Sharing (UNOS) that operates and maintains a computer-assisted organ allocation program that organises the allocation of donated organs to candidates in the national waiting list according to well-defined criteria. When organs become available, several criteria are utilised in identifying the best match organ/recipient(s). The criteria are organised as an index where points are allocated to each candidate, and the selected candidate is the patient with the highest number of points on the index. Kidney points are given by blood type match and histocompatibility (tissue type, number of antigen matches; sensitisation points (PRA) (see note 95); age if under 18); and length of time on the waiting list and medical urgency. Preference is given to recipients with highest priority from the same geographic area as the donor, so as to avoid excessive transportation delays (Annual Report of the Scientific Registry of Transplant Recipients, 1995). The organ harvesting is organised through local Organ Procurement Organisations (OPOs).

UNOS, like Eurotransplant, is an excellent example of a technically sophisticated system with high transparency (of the rules and procedures) as well as high routinisation and predictability. This reduces the chances of suspicions arising that the system shows favouritism, allocates organs in an arbitrary way, or, in general, makes unfair judgements. The fact that the factors and factor weightings are not identical and that they have different default rules point up the variation between allocation systems.

Even in the USA system,[95] as Dennis et al. (1991: 10-11) emphasises, four out of five kidneys are distributed at the regional level of the OPO, and, therefore, the aim to establish a centralised, large waiting list is partially frustrated. There are many OPOs that choose to use point systems which de-emphasise HLA matching and therefore one of the main reasons to establish a single centralised waiting list. Some in the USA advance the argument, as in Spain, that local primacy advantages procurement. UNOS has, nevertheless, a mandatory sharing rule for perfectly-matched kidneys. Every recovered kidney for which there is a zero-mismatch with a potential receiver must be offered to the transplant centre caring for the patient, regardless of the distance between donor and recipient (Dennis, 1991:11). Within UNOS there is great diversity in the ways that kidney waiting lists are constructed in multi-centre organ procurement organisations: some OPOs operate with single lists (more than half (56%) of the 54 multi-centre OPOS do so). All local transplant candidates are on the OPO-wide waiting list. Procured kidneys are distributed to patients with the highest scores on the OPO list. Kidney distributions are made without consideration of which centre cares for a patient to be transplanted. Procurement teams expect to "keep none" (Dennis, 1991:15). Some OPOs are multi-list systems (24%).

Each transplant centre in the OPO maintains its own waiting list. Kidney allocations are made from the lists of each particular centre. Rights to procurement between centres are distributed by a rotation rule. Procurement teams expect to keep two kidneys (Dennis, 1991:15). 20% of the OPOs combine the two systems, by keeping one procured kidney and sharing the second (as Scandiatransplant and France Transplant). There is an OPO-wide list at the same time that each centre maintains its own list. Each and every transplant centre "keeps" the first procured kidney. This is distributed by the local centre according to its own list and the second is shared and distributed by the OPO in accordance with its list.

Similar to Scandiatransplant's policy, UNOS emphasises reciprocity and payback. Thus, when a kidney is voluntarily shared together with an organ other than a kidney from the same donor into the same recipient, the OPO receiving the kidney is supposed to offer through UNOS a kidney from the next suitable donor of the same ABO blood type as the donor from whom the shared kidney was procured. Similarly, for the payback of kidneys shared for highly sensitised recipients: when a kidney is voluntarily shared because the patient for whom it is offered has a PRA of 80% or greater and a negative preliminary crossmatch with the donor, the OPO receiving the kidney shall offer through the UNOS Organ Centre, a kidney from the next suitable donor of the same ABO blood type as the donor from whom the shared kidney was procured.

Multiple Criteria and Dilemmas of Selection

Due to the scarcity of organs for transplantation and the very high costs of transplantation, a number of criteria of selection and prioritisation are established to guide the selection of recipients. Some of the selection criteria are strictly medical; others, possibly related to medical criteria, are of a much more obvious social and psychological character. The selection of suitable candidates for transplantation is regarded as one of the main factors in the success of transplantations. Experience with the application of criteria to concrete cases contributes to later adjustments and reformulations of criteria in selection rules and protocols.

As I indicated earlier, the process of selection of patients for kidney transplantation entails a process that initially starts at the level of a physician in charge, often at a local dialysis unit. Thus, physicians at local dialysis units are often responsible for a pre-transplantation assessment and referral of her/his patient to a transplantation program. The prioritisation and ultimate selection of recipients takes place at the transplantation centre – following the rules of organ exchange and allocation agencies such as Eurotransplant, Scandiatransplant, or UNOS in the USA, or the rules of local transplant centres in Spain or Scandinavia. This is "selection proper". The various criteria in prioritising patients and making selections of recipients entail combinations of medical, quasi-medical, and non-medical criteria: cross-matching organ/patient, health status including emergency status, patient immunisation (a common allocation criterion concerns "sensitised" patients, patients that require a high degree of match), and individual waiting time. Even organisational criteria (exchange requirements among units) and psycho-social criteria play a role. Let us examine these in more detail.[96]

Biomedical Criteria[97]

Biomedical admission criteria: These include factors that have an impact on medical feasibility or eventual success of the transplantation. Serious renal dysfunctions are, of course, indicative. Contraindications in most transplant programs are cardiovascular diseases, potentially terminal cases of cancer, serious chronic pulmonary diseases, HIV-positive patients or old age (for example some programs establish an upper limit for kidney transplantation at 75 years), that is, systemic factors that affect survival or rehabilitation. Biomedical criteria are generally regarded the most "neutral" ones, and the ones most often and consistently stressed in the selection of patients for transplantation. Also they are commonly understood to be more accurate, since they better suit premises of measurability and standardisation, but in daily medical practice, biomedical criteria often merge with other type of criteria.

Biomedical prioritisation criteria: The main biomedical factors in the prioritisation of candidates are: (1) blood type compatibility; (2) good tissue compatibility between graft organ and recipient. This is the most important applied criteria in the selection of candidates, but has the disadvantage of excluding those groups in the population with rare antigens (often minorities). Also, the importance given to high tissue match between patient and graft organ varies among transplantation physicians. The risk of a less than perfect matching has to be weighed in relation to physical deterioration of the patient's health, as she waits for a transplant; (3) highly sensitised patients have priority if tissue typing shows high compatibility between those patients and a donated organ. These are potential recipients with unusual antigens, or patients sensitised as a result of a long waiting time in dialysis, or in retransplantation (increasing the risk for rejection of the graft organ); (4) urgency: the urgency factor based on medical criteria gives priority to the most serious cases on the waiting list; (5) body size: the size of the organ must to a greater or lesser extent correspond to the size of the body of the recipient.

Psychosocial Criteria

Psychosocial criteria are mainly taken into account as contraindicating factors to the admission of patients into a transplantation program, but can also become prioritisation indicators in the choice of recipients. These criteria are diffuse and their application depends on the interpretation of the physicians but they generally relate to the level of self-discipline and cooperation on the part of the candidate. Serious psychosocial problems are regarded as highly problematic since they can jeopardise a transplantation, e.g. inability to follow the often lifelong post-transplantational medicine regimes. Serious "psychosocial problems" cannot be understood out of the moral/sociocultural context in which they appear. However, in principle, a history of mental disease or abuse of substances are often taken into account. Enough psychological stability is regarded as an important factor due to the patient's long convalescence period and strict medicine regime after transplantation.[98] Psychosocial difficulties are not only negative indicators. Some may function as informal "urgency" criteria related to contingent medical or psychological situations. An example of this is the prioritisation of patients with increasing problems of adaptation to dialysis or psychic hardships associated with waiting on a transplantation list.

Normative Criteria

Two common ethical principles concern equity, that is distributive justice, and effective utility, that is making good use of the organs for as many people as possible. One could select recipients randomly as in a lottery – this would maximise even-handedness. However, it would be offensive to many patients (and next-of-kin as well as possibly authorities and politicians) in that it would not assure that organs go to those most in need. Some with less need would obtain organs, while those in urgent need might have to wait. This can be seen as unjust. Many systems have waiting lists that take into consideration how long a potential recipient has been waiting. A system giving priority to the patient who has waited long might be judged to be basically fair (that is adherence to a "first come, first served" principle). But giving the organs to patients most in need would also be judged to be fair or equitable – and would be *unrelated* to length of waiting time. In general, several different principles of justice may be applied and imply different, sometimes contradictory, approaches to allocation.

In Eurotransplant and the UNOS systems, HLA matching has been given considerably more weight than waiting time, but the increased effectiveness of immunosuppressors, an average of low points in most matches, the medical advantages of allocating the kidney locally (avoiding long distance transportation and ischemic damage) and the unintended discriminatory effect that matching criteria has had for racial minorities (with unusual antigens to match) has resulted in policy reflections and changes in the USA. Today the UNOS system assigns more weight to waiting time in order to improve the chances of recipients with difficult matches. Still this is a highly debated area together with the issue of retransplantation. Retransplant patients are often given priority over other candidates. Since primary transplantation has a higher rate of efficacy than retransplantation, it is also a matter of debate whether it is fair to allow individuals to receive multiple transplants. In this particular case, non-medical considerations are taken into account, such as the special obligations that transplant teams feel in not abandoning patients on whom they have already grafted an organ.

A further criterion – based on a principle of *institutional equity* – consists in maintaining a fair distribution of services for all local hospitals of a region. For example, in Sweden each one of the five transplantation centres in the country covers an appointed region, thus providing services for all the inhabitants in their respective regions. The Uppsala region covers 22 hospitals, and the University hospital where the transplantation unit is located. A fair distribution of services in the region also implies taking into account those hospitals that have not received services in a long time.[99]

Discussion and Conclusions

This brief examination of organ allocation suggests several patterns and issues:

(1) The diversity of allocation models – there is no single, universal model – is perhaps surprising. One might have expected in an area of high technology and advanced scientific medicine the emergence of a scientifically based system for allocating organs. Even among highly rationalised national systems, such diversity can arise as well (as in Sweden, France (Dennis et al., 1991), Spain, or the USA).

(2) There are multiple moral imperatives, and different systems put their emphases differently. A centralised system such as Eurotransplant puts the stress on effectivity and abstract concepts of justice, including taking into account those who may be geographically (or otherwise) disadvantaged. Spain, in contrast, puts the emphasis on local "community" and its particular allocative mechanisms as well as potentialities for procuring organs. (Of course, such an arrangement also converges with the interests of local transplant surgeons and other professionals who want to do their best for their own patients (as well as possibly advance their own local careers).)

(3) There is, nonetheless, a certain common denominator in most organ allocation systems: the dimensions of blood type and antigen compatibility as well as hyper-immunological sensitivity.[100] Often a number of additional other quasi- or even non-medical factors are taken into account, for example how long patients have been waiting for a transplant, or how generous or effective their hospital or transplant centre has been in providing organs for others.

(4) A major distinction, as indicated above, is between highly centralised allocation systems (Eurotransplant) and decentralised systems (Spanish National Transplant), or mixtures of these as in the case of Scandiatransplant, France Transplant, and UNOS. The centralised systems are typically formalised (otherwise, they run the risk of being perceived as distant, arbitrary or inscrutable authorities, potentially damaging local procurement capacity; hence, explicit and transparent rules are formalised in point systems). Scandiatransplant and France Transplant, in particular, try to balance local needs with global necessities, by specifying rules of allocation at the global level, but allowing diversity at the local level. For instance, each transplant centre in Scandinavia has its own allocation rules. In France also, the

local transplant centre has discretion in its selection of recipients (Dennis et al., 1991: 10).

But why centralise, in the face of local or regional opposition. The prevalence of large centralised, formalised systems can be traced to the conceptions established from the start, in the case of kidney transplants, that histocompatibility is all important. From this perspective the larger the pool, the better the chances to achieve a compatible match between patient and receiver (Matesanz and Miranda, 1996). An argument advanced in the USA is that "to the extent technically achievable, *any* citizen or resident in the territory of the USA in need of a transplant should be considered as a potential recipient of each retrieved organ on a basis equal to that of a patient who lives in the area where the organs or tissues are retrieved" (Dennis, 1991:9). This principle stresses a universal procedural or formal equality (Dennis, 1991:9), ignoring, however, problems with the transportation of organs. Or with the loyalties and commitments to a local or regional network.

Even in the case of a purely medical criterion such as HLA compatibility, there is some disagreement about the relative importance of matching. For example, UNOS and Eurotransplant stress this factor whereas the Spanish central network (ONT) does not. The proponents argue, as indicated above, that matching should be used for the optimisation of the selection of kidney recipients: the better the match, the better the expected medical outcome. Since the proportion of patients satisfying a high matching of kidney and recipient increases with the size of recipient waiting lists, advocates of HLA matching favour centralising waiting lists. Sceptics of tissue typing judge that advances in immunosuppressive therapy and other factors are equally or more important, and see no substantial medical need for centralising most waiting lists. In Spain, HLA compatibility is considered of relatively minor importance (Spain, 1996:48). On the other hand, the Spanish put a stress on the problems of organ procurements and believe that a decentralised system with local waiting lists is most effective at this. Moreover, decentralised organisations have the advantage of closely connecting the local donor and also the local recipient. It also promotes efficiency in allowing for each local transplantation centre to utilise their own particular resources to solve their particular problems. However, the question remains of the extent decentralised systems allow for a satisfactory level of accountability and fairness concerning organ allocation in a larger perspective.[101]

In developing its procurement, co-ordination and allocation system (OTS), Spain has particularly emphasised the problems of organ shortages and the need to organise in ways to optimise procurement. Matesanz and Miranda (1996) point out the importance of "local altruism" and the evidence from the USA of the inverse relationship between size of OPO and the donation rates achieved. They (1996:50) write: "Every community has its own characteristics, not only are decisions different but also the distribution of resources. The latter is better made at a local level however necessary it is to have a centrally co-ordinated course of action. Centralised decisions, although quite simple for organ distribution, are often experienced as something detached and are a source of strong centrifugal tensions." In short, priority is given to local and regional utilisation, leaving national co-ordination to focus on special programs of hyperimmunised patients, children, and organs without local recipient. In general, the national co-ordination centre takes care of difficult, often rare, cases.

(5) The main types of organ allocation criteria discussed above notwithstanding, who gets an organ (i.e. how these criteria are combined in the choices made) also depends on factors other than particular formal or informal guidelines: the amount of organ donors available, the standard applied to evaluate suitability of the graft organs, the available transplantation centres in a country, the possibility of multiple patient listing, competition between centres in the a country for resources, size and experience of the particular organisation etc. Also a variety of contingencies and ad-hoc factors affect the determination of who obtain organs: individual perception of disease, even individual characteristics such as a patient being too shy or not sufficiently articulated will affect his/her position in a prioritisation queue. And external structural factors can be mentioned such as a physician's capacity to detect end-stage kidney failure in rural communities, the general belief or disbelief in transplant in the medical community, public opinion and political and economic considerations. Since the organisation of the OTS is commonly subject to policy discussions regarding, for example, the efficiency of having few or many centres or increased access to funds, the pressures to achieve *good results is not negligible*. A minimising risk option is to choose "likely-to-succeed patients", restricting selection in order to optimise the results of the transplantation.[102] This, of course, biases access to transplants, but this is true of most expensive medical treatments.

   OTS designers try to cope, of course, with supply and demand imbalances. This is done in part through reformulating laws (e.g. some believe that presumption of consent legislation facilitates the acquisition of organs for transplantation), and conditions of donation criteria (even 70 year olds may now contribute), as well as reformulating criteria for recipient selection or donation procedures (e.g. the distribution of donor cards among the population). Other legal measures often considered are mandatory donation requests in the hospital, and/or mandatory donor referral to the transplantation program. However, the results obtained by the Spanish ONT point at the importance of focusing on organ procurement, in other words, having the problem of the supply/demand imbalance as a central organisational consideration.

(6) Systems such as Eurotransplant and UNOS with algorithmic allocation procedures (based on point systems) give decidability or decisiveness in the selection process. Time need not be devoted to complex discussions, weighings, negotiations – except initially in setting up the protocol. Hence, *transaction costs are reduced*. The mechanical or algorithmic allocation, once agreed upon, may qualify as a type of procedural fairness or justice in that it pre-empts the uneven or arbitrary application of selection criteria (Dennis et al., 1991). In general, formalised procedures assure that arbitrary criteria, or possibly morally objectionable criteria, are not applied (such as selection on the basis of gender, race, social status, religion, political beliefs). They tend to be rigid and impersonal in the face of a complex and ambiguous reality. The designers and users of such algorithms may easily fall into the trap of presuming that they have captured reality in their formulas, and also have effectively addressed ethical issues and predicaments. That is, there is a great risk of losing reflectivity, particularly moral reflectivity, and the meta-imperative for such reflection and discourse.

5 Structural Incongruence

Introduction: Social Relationships in the OTS

The process of transplantation is one in which numerous actors in different roles are co-ordinated, and regulated through administrative and exchange structures. The actors operate under particular laws and regulations, and are co-ordinated by means of specific institutional arrangements. Such a system is an amalgamation.[103] Components do not necessarily fit well together. Some may operate as bottlenecks, limiting or preventing the full effectiveness or efficient operation of the system (Hughes (1983) refers to "reverse salients"). Often there are tensions and conflicts between participating groups and individuals representing different perspectives and professional or social interests. Such conflicts may concern, for instance, the shift from cardio-respiratory death criteria to more "indirect" ones such as brain death, or the appropriateness of asking grieving next-of-kin to authorise the organ donation from a deceased relative.

One of the main problems of organising any complex social system – particularly large-scale and high-tech systems such as the OTS – is that *different social and physical structures must be linked together into a more or less integrated, functioning or operative whole, at least if the system is to perform effectively*. Legal and other social and political demands must be more or less integrated with technical-medical demands.[104]

Organisational Co-ordination

In the organisation of OTS, several organisational forms operate within an overarching network organisation. Administrative co-ordination regulates the physicians' and nurses' activities. Network co-ordination operates in the procurement of cadaveric organs for transplantation (a key input in the organisation). The extractions and implantations are organised and carried out within the organisational frame of a hospital.

The synchronisation of different organisational forms in the OTS creates problems of structural tension at the interface between diverse units of the organisation. These organisational tensions become manifest as organisational incongruencies, reflected in "issues", for example problems and tensions relating to "brain death", organ procurement, organ request or the selection of recipients. Different organisational values and views of the world confront one another, generating tensions and unstable conditions.

Hierarchy and Formalisation as Underlying Dimensions

In order to identify and understand the structural sources of tension in the OTS, one must differentiate basic types of relationships operating in complex organisations such as the OTS. Various types of relationships are structured on the basis of two distinct dimensions, *hierarchisation* and *formalisation*. Variation in the degree of hierarchisation and formalisation of the main social relationships in the organisation of OTS clusters these relationships in several basic mechanisms of co-ordination: (a) administrative co-ordination (formal rules and vertical relationships), (b) formal market or contractual type co-ordination (formal rules and horizontal relationships), and (c) network co-ordination (based on informal rules with either horizontal or vertical relations) (see Table 10).

Table 10. Typology of organisational relationships

	Vertical Modes	**Horizontal Modes**
Formalised	Administrative relationships ① ②	Market and contractual relationships ③ ④ ⑤
Non-formalised	Collegial and professional networks ⑥	Status relations in networks ⑦ ⑧

Organisational theorists increasingly refer to three types of social organisations: hierarchy or bureaucracy, markets, and networks (or clans in Ouchi (1991)) (Nohria and Eccles, 1992; Thompson et al., 1991; Wellman and Berkowitz, 1988). My typology, in contrast, stresses the underlying social relations and constitutive rules, and the fact that *these organisational relationships are not fully compatible*. In this approach, the different contents of relationships are conceptualised and made understandable in terms of the different rules and grammars for constituting and regulating relationships. In a word, they have different rationalities or logics (Burns and Flam, 1987; Burns and Dietz, 1996). In the following paragraphs I briefly describe the different types of relationships and particular variants that occur in the OTS.

I. Administrative Relationships

Administrative relationships are characterised by relations of superordination and subordination (hierarchy), formalisation of rules, specialisation of function, objective qualifications and qualities of office, patterning behaviour according to a fixed set of formal or explicit rules, and differentiation of complex tasks into discrete sub-tasks (Burns and Flam, 1987:216-219; Frances et al., 1991:10; Scott, 1981:68-71; Weber, 1968). In the OTS, at least two different types of such relationships can be identified:

① *Hospital-ward organisation*: this is an administrative form, organised in specialised tasks and functions, and hierarchically structured (Fox, 1989).

② *Physician-patient relationship*: Physician-patient relationships in hospital settings are, from a structural perspective, formal and hierarchical.[105] They are formal in the sense that the duties and responsibilities of physicians and other medical personnel are explicitly formulated (in laws, and hospital and professional association policies) in relation to the care of their patients.[106] Relationships between physicians and patients are hierarchical since physicians have the responsibility and authority to determine what is the best treatment to help their patients.[107]

II. Market and Contractual Relationships

A market is a particular type of social organisation or structure that enables buyers and sellers to come together and defines and regulates their interactions (Burns, 1995; Burns and Flam, 1987: Chapters 8 and 9; Thompson, 1991).[108] Markets as other types of social organisations and relationships are constituted and regulated by systems of shared social rules. A normative and institutional order – laws, group and community norms, and conventions – operate to structure and regulate market entry (who participates, who is excluded), transaction forms and procedures, where and when market activities or transactions are to take place.

Market and contractual relations are largely non-hierarchical in character. This type of relationships is sustained by a rationality of co-ordination based on the voluntary exchange of goods or services between two parties (at agreed and known prices). Market relationships are characterised by decentralised decision-making with participants pursuing their self-interests (Thompson et al., 1991:9).

Market type rules may vary, from the most formal variant such as those defining the proper form(s) of contracts between partners, to the less formal variant as in illegal markets, where at least the buyer and the seller both know what is being bought and sold and the agreed price. The formal aspect of market relationships appears not so much in its core exchange structure as in the determination of limits.[109]

Rules of contract are never exhaustive. Transactions are supported by extra-market rules (for example, those underlying trust), unless very simple items are exchanged (implying that market exchange of complex items as well as labour markets would be difficult to arrange without a well-developed normative and legal order).

Some of the formal rules and regulations defining modern market transactions are clearly stipulated in the regulation of important goods (e.g. quality controls of food or electrical appliances) and in the restriction of some critical goods, etc. (Burns and Flam, 1987: Chapter 9). Informal rules are the result of a market operating in a social context with informal moral boundaries (widespread cultural conceptions of what are socially acceptable as commodities or "marketable" goods).

In the OTS, the following market and contractual relationships may be identified:

Markets

③ *Market provision of technical/pharmaceutical/non-medical resources and services necessary in organ transplantation*: These services and resources are provided through external suppliers as well as through internal markets. The latter are market-like relationships internal to the health care services.

④ *Buying and selling of organ transplantation services*: For example, in the Swedish OTS this is a contractual relation between hospitals where market rules prevail (price competition), it works as an internal market to the health care services (in Sweden transplant services cannot be sold to private individuals on a market external to the health care system). In contrast, the US system has a great internal variation since people with permanent kidney failure requiring transplants can be financially covered personally or under national insurance systems such as Medicare, Medicaid or private insurances (National Transplant Assistance Fund, 1998).

Contractual Relationships

⑤ *Organ donation to unrelated recipients*: Individuals can sign donation cards. This formally (potentially) couples them to the health care system, in other words they enter into a type of contractual relationship where, in the eventuality of death, the system may make use of the person's body parts for transplantation purposes.[110]

III. Network Relationships

The network concept refers to informal relationships between social agents and agencies. These can emerge and operate on the basis of friendship, kinship or ethnic relationships. In the business world, one finds the informal idea of trading partners and business contacts and networking (as opposed to a formal contractual relations). Professional and elite groups often form networks – on the basis of sharing a common outlook and normative understandings – and can discuss and decide policy informally between themselves (Frances et al., 1991:14). In general, network relationships are relatively permanent non-formalised relationships, vertical as well as horizontal, between social actors. As an instance of egalitarian relationships, the collegiate organisation is a classic example (Frances et al., 1991:14). However, among academics, for instance in a hospital or medical school, the physicians are differentiated in prestige and status, in some cases irrespective of the formal positions they hold. Patron-client networks may also be hierarchical, but typically non-formalised in character.

Networks tend to emerge outside of and within the interstices of formal social relations. They are in the form of more or less established friendship ties, kin relationships, business partnerships, professional ties etc. Political elites and professional groups often form networks based on a common ethical outlook. The co-ordination of networks is not always overtly open to accountability (Thompson et al., 1991:14). In contrast to bureaucracies and markets, the central co-ordination mechanism is personal or professional trust and cooperation. In the OTS, the following types of networks are prominent:

Professional Networks[111]

Uniform networks and multi-professional networks linking professions of different types.

⑥ *Physician-physician peer relations not included in* ①: these are non-formalised professional networks that combine informal peer relationships (Fox, 1959; Bidwell, 1976). This is often key to the mobilisation of expertise or other strategic resources. Such informal, egalitarian peer relationships are observable in the frequent professional consultations in order to deal with health problems of patients that are not administratively regulated (Coleman and Katz, 1957).

⑦ *Professional status relations*: informal status relationships, that is relations of higher or lower status and prestige among physicians (or other professional groups) are established in the course of clinical work and research (Coleman and Katz, 1957). These differences are based on professional achievements, recognition, demonstrations of expertise.

Mixed Networks

⑧ *Professional/non-professional contacts*: Medical personnel meet next-of-kin and friends of patients in relatively non-formalised ways. There may also be formal aspects when, for example, the relative of a patient becomes the legal guardian. The relationship is a vertical one because of the status of medical professionals, and because the interaction takes place in medical contexts, where the non-professionals not only lack expertise but are unfamiliar with the (hospital) order and somewhat outside the social structure of the hospital units whereas patients become a part of the structure (concerning this notion see Anspach (1993)).

In sum, the social organisation of organ transplantation entails a number of *different but highly interdependent activities/processes* where different actors are co-ordinated and interact. Complex organisations other than OTS present similar characteristics of tight coupling, interdependence, scarcity of resources and variability in the input flow (Perrow,1979), but in the OTS these features are particularly highlighted because of culturally and emotionally "laden" issues that the system's activities raise: the use of the bodies of the dead.

In the following section, I will apply my own approach to identifying and analysing structural incongruence and tension within complex organisations such as OTS.

Incongruence and Tensions Between Organisational Relationships

Complex social organisations such as OTS are characterised by *heterogeneous relationships*.[112] The various relationships imply different *normative orders*. Cleavages and tensions are generated at the interfaces between different types of relations. In the organisational literature on complexity, there is some recognition that combining heterogeneous relationships, such as those of bureaucracy, market, and network, cannot be accomplished without problems (Thompson et al., 1991; Nokria and Eccles, 1992; Powell, 1990; Wellman and Berkowitz, 1988). But typically the problems are seen as co-ordination problems, technical or managerial (in a limited sense) in character, or differences in professional and occupational perspectives. It is rare that organisational researchers identify the problems in terms of structural bases – also normative in character – of incongruence, tension and conflict. However, some authors suggest, without actually employing such a concept, that zones of incongruence occur in organisational structures, and that at these points behaviour will be less predictable or orderly (DiMaggio, 1992:132). Moreover, these structural conditions may interfere with or block the capacity of the organisation and its members to act effectively (unless particular ways are found to deal with such problems). In sum, my main point is that the heterogeneous relationships, when put together, are not the same as combining material components. Each relationship has its own modality and logic, its underlying rule system which orients and regulate the actors adhering to them. Interfaces between different types of relationship become zones of incongruence and tension. Recognising this enables one to address and understand the problems more effectively.

Important foci of structural tension in the OTS result from: (a) patterns of incongruence between types of social relationships that interface or converge in the OTS; (b) particular decision-making situations characterised by unclear or contradictory rules within the social organisation.

Organisational incongruity implies contradictory orientations and tensions in the sense that the two rule systems constituting and regulating particular relationships cannot be applied simultaneously to the same situation: for example administrative rules, on the one hand, and network rules on the other. Administrative requirements of predictability cannot be met by the network character of the social organisation; nor does administrative rationality fit professional rationality.

While structural tensions emerge as the result of greater or lesser incompatibility in rule systems, tensions associated with particular decision-making settings are the result of unclarity about which rules to apply and disagreements about who has the right or competence to decide about them. A common source of problems arises *from unclarity about which jurisdiction the situation concerns*, that is which actors, procedures and rules are to prevail in decision-making (for instance, who is to decide about the use of organs of a recently deceased when important members of the family disagree). Additional problems arise from instances where the actors in a position of responsibility for a consequential decision do not have enough control and substantial information. For example, even if jurisdictional areas are well defined, such situations arise when OTS physicians (legally responsible) must assess the freedom of choice of an individual donating a kidney – a situation in which particular family pressures can play an important role (Fox and Sweazy, 1974).

Structural Incongruities 1: Tensions Between Networks

Important instances of structural tension in the social organisation of OTS are generated at network interfaces or boundaries between different types of networks. That is, different rule systems are applied in the transactions between networks related to the OTS. For example, in the Swedish OTS, actors in local professional networks, informal organ-sharing networks (as distinct from the formalised, contractual relations established in Eurotransplant and UNOS), and family networks are brought into interaction with one another.

Typically, medical professionals maintain jurisdiction over issues regarded as medically defined areas of authority and competence. Next-of-kin have jurisdiction over decisions defined as family matters. In the encounter between actors in these two networks, competition arises between professional and family jurisdictions, thus opening possibilities for tensions and conflict at the interface (Anspach 1993). For example, a family may object to the medical diagnosis that a patient is "beyond hope", because of their commitment or a particular religious belief that the family advocates. In general, the role of the physician is ambiguous in this interface between the "profane" professional world of medicine and the solidarity, emotional world of a family caring about a sick relative or mourning the deceased. Issues of "futility", mode of treatment, organ request, etc. does not follow the typical patient-physician interaction pattern, with clear procedural boundaries. The next-of-kin of a deceased donor has its own internal rules, obligations and loyalties, and may find it difficult to accept or comply with the demands or expectations of the medical order (e.g., that organs for transplantation and research be extracted from the body of the deceased).

A particularly problematic interface arises in the contact between the next-of-kin and the organ-requesting physicians of ICUs and emergency units in the case of cadaver donation, and between transplantation surgeons and relatives in "living" organ donation.

The organ request interface: The interaction between the organ-requesting physician and the relatives of a recently deceased produces in most cases a difficult situation for both sides (Lowy and Martin, 1992:113). These situations are an instance of structural tension between the network of the next-of-kin with their particular norms and values, and the physicians in a professional network with its own norms and values.

Both the professional and next-of-kin networks may appear structurally similar but their character and constitution differ substantially, entailing different dynamics, alliances, language, scope,[113] power distribution, intensity of ties between their members, and also different (cognitive) jurisdictions.[114] The organ request does not follow the typical patient-physician interaction pattern, where the role of the physician (as well as the patient) is more or less predictable and with clear procedural boundaries. The next-of-kin of a deceased donor has its own internal rules, obligations and loyalties, and does not have to be compliant with the medical order. Since the roles of the interaction are not clearly defined *a situation of ambiguity* is produced (see Chapter 6). In principle, the physician has to shift in his/her role as former helper of the deceased patient, the hierarchy line is also modified since the physician may not be able to exercise her/his professional authority either. As the request for organs in cadaver donations is done almost immediately after the person's death – a very stressful time for the relatives of the deceased – the request can be experienced as awkward by both parties, increasing the tensions of the encounter.

The living donor interface: Living donation involves kin rules concerning mutual help, obligations, etc. For a transplantation surgeon it is very difficult to assess if a decision to donate is a free act of generosity or a consequence of familial pressures. This is particularly important since an organ donor is not a patient, but a healthy individual that will be exposed to a not negligible risk.

The decision of a family member to become an organ donor is often the result of collective decisions or a series of negotiations internal to the family (Fox and Sweazy, 1974), which has jurisdiction over decisions and actions defined as family matters (i.e., family competence). The physician responsible for assessing the suitability of the donor does not have access to much of this information or control over the situation (although he would be held accountable).

Local patients and the rules of organ allocation: Another illustration of incongruence and tensions at network interfaces relates to organ exchange. The exchange of organs between centres organised through the organ-sharing network, is co-ordinated and regulated on the basis of certain rules (i.e. giving priority to particular types of recipients and thus motivating particular allocation of organs). In some instances, the exchange rules of the organ-sharing network come into conflict with the allocation rules of the local centre (as in the case of emergencies, when for example a patient waiting for an organ suddenly deteriorates, and there is a risk that she cannot undergo a transplantation at a later date). Physicians have responsibilities towards their own patients but are to follow the organ-sharing rules (i.e. the larger network priorities conflict with the local network). That is, responsibility towards local patients is a concern of the local medical network.

Responsibility towards patients in other centres and to an efficient allocation of organs are concerns of the key actors in the organ-sharing network. Infraction of these rules is informally disapproved, however no particular administrative or legal sanction has been established for a centre breaking, e.g., exchange rules.[115] The potential incongruity between the rules of the different networks would become a major source of tension if the organ scarcity and eventually the competition for organs increased substantially.[116]

Structural Incongruence 2: Administrative-Network-Market Tensions

An administration organisation is, in a certain sense, not fully congruent with everyday networks where the stress is on flexibility and openness, and where the formalisation, standardisation, and detailed predictability of bureaucracy are not characteristic features. The universalistic rules of the formal organisation tend to clash with the particularistic, flexible rules of, for example, friendship networks (Heimer, 1992).

An obvious source of incongruence and tension concerns the interface of medical personnel adhering to the universalistic, more or less fixed rules of the hospital, its clinics, operating rooms, and various routine tasks, on the one hand, and the particularistic – and widely applicable – rules of family relationships. Fox (1989:147) refers to the incongruence and tensions that arise when the universalistic, "detached concern" of medical personnel is confronted with the profound concerns of next-of-kin in the context of death, dying, and organ extraction.[117] Administrative considerations and procedures in the modern hospital, and "professional detached concern" are a frequent source of dissonance and tension particularly around post-mortem care (Fox, 1989:147). A substantial sociological literature provides accounts of critical, symbolic cases – whether the dying child or youth; the suicidal patient – that bring questions of meaning and moral worth so acutely to the surface that institutionalised rules and procedures for dealing with death temporarily break down, and with them the usual capacity of medical personnel to manage their feelings (Fox, 1988:429).

A further source of incongruence between professions and market forces relates to different moral or ethical perspectives on health and matters of life or death. Medical professions are ill-disposed to putting a price on health or on life-and-death matters. However, market-based health insurance and medical organisations (but also public ones) subject to market rules do just this, calculating costs, gains, and losses. Thus, market or market-like processes may operate to minimise or cut costly procedures and treatments – procedures and treatments which physicians and nurses may consider essential both for medical and ethical reasons. Such incongruence, and related tensions and conflicts, are endemic in contemporary hospitals and clinics.

The case of internal markets and designated harvesting region: Another example – as of now hypothetical in a Swedish context – of administrative-market rule discrepancy is the recently proposed establishment of national markets for the provision of transplantation services (not organs), operating concurrently with administrative configuration of the harvesting regions. The administrative order of the Swedish OTS was designed as an arrangement between estimated transplantation needs, production of services, and size of harvesting regions for each centre (concerning, for example, kidneys). The original design has been modified by the introduction of a market rules (i.e. competition through quality and prices). In principle, patients in need of organs – or more precisely their physicians – apply to any centre in Sweden for a transplantation. A centre providing good results at lower prices could – at least in theory – increase the number of clients and the volume of production, but since the size of the harvesting region remains unchanged, organ supply is constrained at the same time that demand for organs increases. Thus, there could result an imbalanced exchange with other regional or Scandinavian centres. This could result in a breakdown of the original planning.

Structural Incongruence 3: Professional and Bureaucratic "Tension Prone" Relations

Tension arising at the interface between professional and bureaucratic relationships is a well-studied phenomenon in the organisational literature (Blau, 1956; Blau and Scott, 1962).[118] Perrow (1979) and Cockerham (1978) have stressed that relationships organised on a professional basis tend to generate tensions if combined with bureaucratic relationships within the same organisation or unit (Parsons 1964). Thus, an individual may be the administrative supervisor (bureaucratic authority) over another with a higher professional competence but still under the authority of the former. This type of incongruity – typical of hospitals and universities as examples of professional bureaucracies – is a chronic source of tension and conflict.

In the OTS, such tensions are also observable. The Board of Health

(*Socialstyrelsen*) in Sweden has determined which transplantation centres are to carry out what types of transplantation: the aim is to eliminate redundancy and wastage of resources, to increase the overall effectiveness of the OTS. As a consequence, the Gothenburg centre is to conduct heart transplants but not Stockholm or Uppsala. However, these administrative measures come into conflict with the professional concerns and interests of transplantation surgeons who want to expand their professional activities, engage themselves on the forefront of technical advances and research, and to gain in national and international status.

Structural Incongruence 4: Incongruent Task Specialisations

Structural tensions can be internal to a particular set of relationships such as an administrative unit. Tension may be generated by task specialisation where those responsible or engaged in different tasks have different goals and norms (for example, within an administrative order, managerial responsibility can conflict with the particular responsibilities of a specialised staff – a common problem in the dual organisations within hospitals). This type of administrative incongruence in the OTS, generated by goal incongruence, is illustrated by two important organisational tasks in the OTS, organ procurement and organ replacement.

A key linkage in the OTS is in the relationship between intensive care units (as well as emergency units) and the transplantation centre. Both units share the same overall purpose of helping patients, but their particular goals can be regarded as incongruous, since all patients certified as deceased by irreversible collapse of cerebral functions in the ICUs (that is a medical failure in the ICU) are potential organ donors. My research indicates that this is a source of tensions and a potentially conflictive linkage in OTS.

Also, in decision-making and task activities such as selection of recipients, there are pressures – and a sense of responsibility – to take into account different values and concerns. Multiple rule systems are applied in the prioritisation and selection of organ recipients: there are, among the explicit rules we find, medical, administrative, and sociopsychological rules (see Chapter 4). Prioritisation and selection of patients are instances of complex decisions where the combination of different sets of rules (concerning selection) can increase the risk of ad hoc selection or disagreements about priorities.[119] This is a major source of tensions and uncertainty in transplantation units. In general, a common source of problems in decision-making arises where *rules or rule systems of very different character are expected to be taken into consideration.*

Implications and Conclusions

My main point is that complexes of heterogeneous relationships or inter-institutional complexes are problematic, giving rise to tension, conflict, and disorder. Each distinct relationship or organising mode has its own modality and logic, its underlying rule system which orients and regulate the actors adhering to them. Each makes up a type of moral order. Interfaces between different types of relationship become zones of potential incongruence and tension. Such a normative-structural theory of social organisation (based on the concepts of rule system and multiple systems of rules) enables us to identify *zones of incongruence and tension* within any complex social organisation such as an OTS. We have indicated a few such zones.

While different types of relationships can be combined or even integrated into more complex arrangements, typically this cannot be done without problems. Alter and Hage (1993), in their study of service systems (educational, medical, mental health care), report that highly differentiated, complex organisational arrangements are strongly correlated with disharmony and conflict. They (1993, p. 94) write: "complexity and differentiation... means that the range of differently trained workers, different perspectives, and unrealistic expectations will be high, which in turn increases opportunities for conflict and combat". Problems in mixing institutional forms and types of relationships are recognised in some of the organisational literature (Laurence and Lorsch, 1967; Bradach and Eccles 1989; Powell 1990; Stinchcombe 1985).

Administrative hierarchy, interpersonal networks, market, and contract type relations are not necessarily mutually exclusive types of relationships and regulative mechanisms. Empirical studies indicate that different relationships are combinable with each other in a variety of ways within a given complex organisation, e.g. informal interpersonal networks in the context of a formal organisation. Administrative hierarchies display features of markets and markets exhibit traits of hierarchy (Burns and Flam 1987). In view of such mixing, some organisational theorists, for example Eccles and Granovetter (see Powell (1990, p. 267)), question whether distinctions in organisational forms such as market, administrative hierarchy, and network are useful at all, in part because sharp demarcations rarely if at all exist – all forms of human interaction and exchange entail elements of the different forms. However, in our view these distinctions are essential, since they are grounded in different rule systems, types of rational and moral orders. This approach alerts one to the problems and chemistry of heterogeneous or multi-institutional complexes, in particular the patterns of incongruence and tension in concrete organisational contexts (Machado, 1995b).

DiMaggio (1992, p. 132) has suggested, without actually employing such a concept, that zones of incongruence or contradiction occur in organisational structures, and that at these points behaviour will be less predictable or orderly. Moreover, *these structural conditions may interfere with or block the capacity of the organisation and its members to act effectively, unless ways are found to manage or deal with such problems. The effective functioning of any complex organisation requires the co-ordination and harmonisation of incongruous modes of organisation and their realisations in concrete programs and domains of activity.* That is, the structural conditions of incongruence can interfere with or block the capacity of the organisation and its members to act effectively. Interface incongruences are weak points in a complex organisation, entailing potential tension and conflict costs, that can substantially *multiply transaction costs.* This principle is central to my insistence on identifying and investigating particular ways in which structural incongruence and related tensions and conflicts appear and are responded to in complex organisational processes, in part through various integrative mechanisms.[120]

Networks are recognised as contributing to the effectiveness of many formal arrangements and, indeed, in dealing with structural incongruence. They appear, however, to be a paradoxical form of organising, since they both contradict and complement other forms. The key to understanding this apparent paradox is the non-formalised character of networks as opposed to formalised orders. Rules are formed and reformed as well as enforced differently in these contrasting orders. Formal organisations [whether formal hierarchy, market, or democracy] are characterised by centralised, systematic rule formation and rule enforcement, e.g. in the case of laws and administrative regulations. At local points of interaction – where, e.g., actors belonging to the formal organisation encounter actors belonging to other organisations and relationships, the organisation's rules are to be complied with. They are enforced by designated agents monitoring and making use of systematic controls including record-keeping. Of course, formal markets as well as many bureaucracies allow considerable local initiative, negotiations, and settlements, but always *within* the formal frame of fixed and uniform procedural rules specifying how tasks and other specified accts are to be performed.

Laws, regulations, and policy are legislated by designated, authoritative agents (although they may be global in their extension, as in the case of some professional networks). Networks lack systemic rule formation. Rather, they have local, organic rule formation and reformation, local negotiation and enforcement. Similarly there is no global or systemic enforcement. Hence, local solutions to problems may be worked out by adapting rules, negotiating new rules and reaching local agreements. Hence, the great opportunities in networks of adapting to local situations, making use of local good-will and contextualised knowledge [activities which in a formal context may risk being centrally defined and sanctioned as deviant]. New or reformed rules diffuse in networks rather than being promulgated by a central authority or legislative body. Networks cannot, of course, readily solve global problems – for instance those requiring global co-ordination, or to stabilise extended network relationships, that is precisely what formal organisations are highly capable of accomplishing.

Networks are a major ingredient in many of the complex social organisations and inter-institutional complexes which characterise organ transplantation. They also operate as a type of socio-cultural infrastructure for dealing with structural incongruence and resolving potential tensions and conflicts. They can play this role precisely because they are not formalised and institutionalised in purely rational terms. They offer flexibility and a spectrum of potential integrative devices with which to deal with conflicts, tensions, and incoherence. Included here are those special devices which I discuss later, for instance rituals, special non-instrumental discourses, and emergent mediating roles.

Formal organising modes have legitimacy and are defined and regulated in terms of law and explicit, even formalised rule systems. Participants have particular material and ideal interests in the functioning, the status and prestige of their particular institutional order and, therefore, in maintaining, even defending its boundaries. There may also be regulative agencies – and legal demands– requiring defence of the integrity and proper functioning of the organising mode. Most networks are characterised by their non-formalised character. They may entail equal or unequal relationships. But they can tolerate more – additional dimensions – and more obvious contradictions. They operate diffusely, pragmatically, generatively in dealing with local conditions, the need for local interpretations and adaptations. In this way, actors may promote (or subvert) formal values and norms, add flexibility, and sustain "the spirit" behind a formal order.

Network actors may establish and carry out rituals and discourses and play roles that would be inappropriate, even illegal, in more formalised contexts. In other words, a variety of practices may be effective and well-established but outside of, and indeed illegitimate in, the formal arrangements. These are the organic niches in an administrative or legal landscape. Networks are characterised then by their great flexibility, even creativity as actors mobilise and mix different modes, varieties of means (rational as well as and non-rational), all done in ways which are not bound to satisfy strict requirements of "order", of "legitimacy", of "proper accounting", etc. characteristic of the formalised organising modes. This practice entails a genuine organic process operating informally, even backstage or in grey or black zones in relation to formal institutionalised domains.

Networks offer substantial flexibility and openness to deploying and developing conflict-resolving and integrative strategies and, therefore, contribute to minimising transaction costs engendered in complex, formal organisations. Typically, there is a *web of informal social organisation* that carries on *invisible* (often non-rational) mechanisms of integration "outside" of market, bureaucracy, formal democratic arrangements, etc., to a high degree functioning to "oil the wheels" of formal organisations (Barnard, 1938). A wide variety of problems, ambiguities, uncertainties, conflicts and problems of judgements can be effectively addressed in ways that would be inappropriate or even illegitimate formally or publicly. Networks are highly effective and robust – because they are less constrained, more open to negotiation – in reducing transaction costs by minimising the costs of innovations in conflict resolution and integration in heterogeneous organisations. Why then do they simply not replace or completely dominate the formal? In some circumstances or contexts, they apparently do so. The result may be rampant corruption, no rule of law; no formal, public predictability and accountability. Predictability, understanding, and accountability are only for insiders, not for a general public, or one or more publics having rights to monitoring and accountability. One major difficulty of such networks, even highly effective ones, is that of sustaining or establishing legitimacy. Even "rationality" may appear threatened in such a shadowy landscape.

In Chapter 8, I identify and exemplify a variety of organisational mechanisms that operate to minimise the effects of incongruence and dissonance and operate to harmonise and integrate heterogeneous parts of a complex organisation. Mediating roles or actors, ritual, discourse and other institutional strategies play a key part in organisational integration and co-ordination across relationships, and in the reduction or resolution of tensions in complex organisation based on multiple rule systems and distinct normative orders.

Mediating roles and units have a key role in integrating different organising modes and social relationships in a complex, heterogeneous organisation. They establish bridges and negotiate between the distinct modes. Attention has been focused in some of the organisational literature on roles where incumbents experience role conflict, the "man-in-the-middle", for example school superintendents dealing with their teachers, on the one hand, and with the democratically elected school board, on the other (Gross et al., 1958). In general, integrative agents, teams, or subsystems with representatives from each of the various differentiated subsystems are formal devices to enable discussion, solution of mutual problems and resolution of conflicts. Lawrence and Lorsch (1972, p. 344) suggest that orientations of mediating or integrative members or subsystems tend to be "intermediate" between those found in the subsystems they co-ordinate. An effective co-ordinator working between, for example research and sales, could be expected to be *oriented equally toward long-term problems (the requisite long time orientation of researchers) and short-term problems (the requisite short time orientation of sales personnel) and to have an equal concern with market goals and scientific goals.* From Lawrence and Lorsch's studies (1972), it appears that effective integration depends on intermediate orientations with respect to time and goal orientations, task concern versus social concern. Differences in time and goal orientations seemed to cause the most difficulty.

Liaison roles are often created or emerge to help the cooperation and production involving different divisions or departments, in part by dealing with tensions and conflict among them (Scott 1981, p. 247).[121] Such a mediating role in Swedish universities is embodied in, for instance, the head of a department, the prefect, who negotiates between the academics of the department and the university administration, the "bureaucrats". Another case is that of "grassroots bureaucrats" who mediate between their government agency and clients with "messy" demands, particular needs and circumstances that often do not fit the classifications and strategies of the agency. Blau (1955) and Blau and Scott (1962) report on the problems of conflicts between welfare service agencies and their clients. Clients would refuse to abide by the formal rules and the authority of the staff personnel dealing with them, for example opposing referrals to other offices. The professionals mediate between client needs and demands and the expectations and requisites of the bureaucratic agency which they represent, resolving misunderstandings and conflicts. This is one of the most important functions of organisational professionals vis-à-vis clients.

A particularly difficult mediating process in medical organisations concerns the interface or passage between sacred and profane domains in hospital settings, for example with respect to critical issues relating to the dying or dead. It is particularly difficult for physicians to combine or mediate different value and norm systems along with their particular discourses. Physicians are authoritative in scientific terms (this is a major basis for their legitimacy). However, in the contemporary world, they are typically not moral leaders or authoritative ethicists (Machado, 1998). If they engage simultaneously in patient care, organ removal and organ transplantation, they confront a situation where their different responsibilities and duties are contradictory and confusing. In a certain sense, they risk contamination (Fox 1993; Douglas 1966). One common solution is to keep these roles strictly separated and creating mediating roles. One such new role is that of ethicist, common at US hospitals and growing in number in Europe. In general, the successful mediators or liaison actors are those who possess attributes and orientations intermediate to the units they bridge as well as command of important skills and essential technical competence. It is also important that they enjoy high status and influence in the various organisational units that they are mediating (see also Scott 1981, p. 247; Lawrence and Lorsch 1967, pp. 54-83).

In a certain sense, organisational and professional buffers or designs, as well as particular rituals and discourses (see Chapter 8), protect key groups against the full impact of multiple and potentially contradictory and destabilising relationships and experiences (including "truthful" but disconcerting information). These mechanisms serve to stabilise social order. All moral communities share in common that they are held together – and social order maintained – through mechanisms grounded in rituals, special non-rational discourses, and situational structures within groups and organisations. There is a continual production of meaning as well as bias and distortion. In this sense, many medical as well as scientific discourses, rituals and props can be – and are – used in magical or mythical ways (Elias, 1996).

While heterogeneity is a source of "organisational problems" – e.g., increased potentialities of conflict and growing transaction costs – it also gives rise to creativity and innovation. That is, while incongruence and tension associated with highly differentiated organisations may be disruptive and damaging to performance unless recognised and effectively regulated, homogeneity tends to inhibit creativity and innovation by restricting diversity (Ibarra 1992, p. 181). Ibarra, drawing on Kanter (1983, 1988), stresses the importance of social contacts between actors who view the world differently, as a logical prerequisite to seeing ourselves differently and to fostering creativity and innovation. In the case of research and development groups, she (1992, p. 181) points out, "...research groups composed of individuals with diverse academic training and affiliation tend to be more productive than less diverse groups". In sum, heterogeneous types of organisations encourage or enhance creativity, reflectivity, and innovation (Burns and Engdahl, 1998). But these organisations risk high levels of tension, misunderstandings, distrust, conflict and, ultimately, high transaction costs. This chapter has suggested a variety of organisational strategies that may deal with some of these problems. For instance, an organisation may combine heterogeneous, incongruent relationships, together with mechanisms for resolving or regulating resultant organisational tensions and conflict. This "dialectical mode of organisation" (Burns et al., 1997) is characterised by inconsistency and tension, by creativity action, and transformation, rather than by consistency, "rationality", and a fixed, stable order.

6 The Ambiguous Body

Introduction

Modern medicine is characterised by the continual introduction of new technologies and techniques for curing diseases, saving lives, or improving the quality of life. Such innovations have significant unintended consequences, including the emergence of organisational, legal and moral problems. Not only are established values and beliefs challenged. People, including professionals, experience events, actions, situations and developments which do not necessarily fit established ways of categorising, perceiving, judging, and acting. For instance, "life-saving" technologies in intensive care units are utilised today for the maintenance of recently deceased for purposes of organ donation and transplantation. The introduction of such technologies has not only cognitive and normative implications but real consequences for medical practice. An important example of this was the establishment of brain-death criteria in defining death. In this case, the improvement and widespread use of the electroencephalograph (previously used in rare cases to certify death), of life-support systems (the ventilator; cardiac defibrillation; feeding tubes), in connection with advances in organ transplantation surgery, led to a reconsideration of the traditional medical criteria for defining death, and to the establishment of a new legal frame for the use of human organs and tissue for therapy and research.[122]

The changes in the legislation and clinical implementation of brain-death challenged and undermined traditional conceptions of death, and also many rules and practices associated with the "appropriate" treatment of the dead. The re-definition of death as the irreversible cessation of cerebral functions (of the brain stem or alternatively of the whole brain) is still debated and an open issue, for example the question of whether or not to define as dead anencephalic new-borns or patients in a permanent vegetative state.[123]

The application of the criteria of irreversible brain failure in defining death builds on advanced technology and expert knowledge, contrasting with everyday notions of death. People still tend to associate death with the "lifeless" cold body lacking bodily signs of life, not with a warm, breathing, perspiring braindead person (Pelletier, 1992). Since the dividing line between a dying and a braindead "patient" is not clear cut for most people, it is difficult for the families of some deceased to accept such diagnosis, particularly when for purposes of transplantation the deceased is actively monitored in the intensive unit and, if necessary, subject to cardiopulmonary "resuscitation".

Most transplantation services depend on access to cadaveric organs for transplantation, that according to current practices are mostly obtained from braindead donors. So far, organ procurement has not been an easy task. Confusion in the public about the concept of brain-death is well known. People are not eager to write donation cards, nearly half of the relatives refuse to approve donation. Many physicians show reluctance to request organs. These are among some of the problems commonly reported with respect to organ procurement (De Vita et al., 1993a).[124] Also the personnel involved with these cases at the intensive and emergency units – familiar with death and dying – have also expressed concerns about caring for braindead. Many of these problems are explained as problems of educating the public and the professionals, and as expressions of irrational thinking.

Thus, medical professionals and the public alike are confronted with new problem situations, new patterns of action, and an existing repertoire of solutions to problems which do not fit with those traditional social rules regarding death on which they have previously relied. This has set the stage for greater or new types of ambiguity as well as increased likelihood of cognitive disturbance or dissonance (see Chapter 7). It should not come as a surprise that brain-death is a very difficult concept for many people to assimilate since it implies important changes in cultural and social understandings about death and bodies.

A basic premise of the following discussion is that classification systems, in particular those relating to human bodies and to matters of life and death, are of profound significance in social life (Douglas 1987, Durkheim 1915, Zerubavel 1993). I stress that the importance of correctly classifying or defining a person as dead or alive resides mainly *in the consequences of such a definition for action toward that person.* To act toward an alive person in the same manner as if she were dead entails a gross disrespect and even moral and legal violation of that person. The braindead are problematic because, while legally dead, they are not assigned unequivocally and completely to the category of dead by some medical personnel and by many next-of-kin. To extract their organs is regarded by most medical personnel as permissible both legally and morally, but only for purposes of helping another person. But the thought of, for example, cremating a braindead with sustained circulation and breathing would be regarded by most as revolting.

A basic model[125] which I develop and illustrate in this chapter is the following:[126] [127]

Technological developments   such as organ transplantation and those related to brain-death, have affected central concepts, values, norms and rituals concerning death, and the human body within medical settings. In defining death by the absence of neurological activity, a situation characterised by multiple meanings is created, or even unclarity: "What's going on here" becomes   ambiguous or unclear, although the opposite is supposed to be the case, given the substantial scientific knowledge mobilised and applied in these settings.[128] Also "high-tech death" sets up a situation where death appears more and more to be a matter of discretion or human determination rather than a natural event. Since specialised competence in the diagnosis is required, the next-of-kin can only roughly judge or verify the judgement by themselves.   The   braindead   (donors)   bodies   are   handled   in unconventional ways and may even appear to be alive and even to experience pain (as some relatives believe).

Figure 8. Changes in bodily conceptions

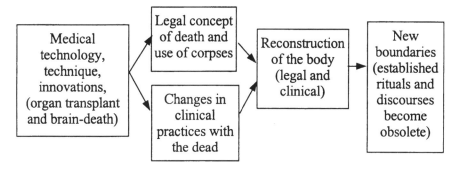

The Clinical Re-construction of the Body

Most transplantation services depend on access to cadaveric organs for transplantation (most often obtained from braindead donors).[129] The determination of death by the criterion of   "total failure of brain functions" has been subject to several controversies inside and outside the medical profession (Horton and Horton, 1991:1048; De Vita and Snyder, 1993:136; De Vita, Snyder and Gränvik, 1993;113-129; Veatch,1993), particularly in connection with organ transplantation surgery. However, important reasons for these controversies are to be found less in the scientific issues *per se* than in the cultural, social and organisational implications of redrawing the line between the living and the dead.

The criteria for establishing that brain-death is the total cessation of all functions seems to offer, like the cardiopulmonary criteria, crystal-clear means for separating the living from the dead. But its application in practice is less clear-cut. As Veatch (1993:18) [130] observes:

> When the uniform definition of death said all functions of the entire brain must be dead, there was a gentlemen's agreement that cellular level functions did not count... This willingness to write off cellular level functions is more controversial than it may appear. After all the law does not grant a dispensation to ignore cellular level functions, no matter how plausible that may be... By 1977 a analogous problem arose regarding electrical activity.

The implementation of brain-death criteria in establishing a new classification of death disrupts in several ways established procedures, rituals and discourses in medical wards relating to life and death. It raises new ethical dilemmas and predicaments. The braindead must be handled in ways which do not fit with established ways of thinking and acting in hospitals. Important reasons for such disruption are:

(a) The determination of death based on neurological criteria – to many neurologists more scientifically accurate than the cardiac/respiratory cessation criteria – requires for its diagnosis a specialised competence in the physician. That is, an adequate level of knowledge and skill are critical. This characteristic increases the importance of expert judgement, in other words increases the *discretionary power* of the diagnosticing physician. Thus, it can easily appear as precariously close to a "deed" (contrary to traditional notions of death as a more "natural event"),[131] particularly in ambiguous situations. This explains the reported incertitude of some relatives of organ donors and even among nurses about whether or not the patient is in fact dead (Fulton et al., 1977:354; Arnold and Youngner, 1993:263-278; Pelletier, 1992; Youngner et al., 1989:2205; Sophie et al., 1983:261; Fernandez et al., 1991:1799-1801). For example, Youngner (1988:356) points out:

> Their decision to allow donation and the cessation of the machines is an irreversible one, while the condition of the heart beating cadaver appears capable of being reversed despite the physician's assurance to the contrary.

(b) Defining death upon the absence of neurological signs implies abandoning the concept of death (i.e. heartbeat and respiration) but also the concept of a "moment" of death (Fox et al., 1993). Although from a legal perspective, death is a moment in time, in brain-death the processual character of death becomes more manifest, since no precise moment of death can be determined (something extending both forward and backward from the moment of a verbal declaration). This explains some of the confusion regarding firmly established cultural conceptions about the moment of death even among health care personnel (Crosby and Waters (1972) in Simmons et al., 1977:28; Fulton et al., 1977: 354-356; Fox et al., 1991; Veatch, 1993; Dominguez et al., 1992:25-26). Pelletier (1992) describes:

> For seven family members, parting with the loved one before the organ/tissue retrieval was begun generated unanswered questions and unresolved doubts about death. One spouse said, "Not being able to be with him [her husband] until he was actually dead was the hardest thing. That's the big thing: I really don't know when T. died.

An even greater problem with the term "brain-death", arises, from the latent doubt that individuals with brain-death are really dead. Hence, not only patients but also nurses and physicians are heard to say that the patient "suffered brain-death" one day and "died" the following day (Pelletier, 1992).

(c) The introduction of procedures to keep a dead patient "functioning" until the "alive" organs can be removed creates a conceptual differentiation between organs and patient. In praxis, this differentiation can be barely maintained, only with great difficulty – both cognitively and normatively – by the personnel in charge of these cases. This lead to ambiguous and dissonant situations. Such situations create concerns associated, for example, with the care of "heart beating cadavers" in intensive care units (Fox, 1993:223; Horton and Horton, 1991:1048; Irwin, 1986:305-310; Sanner, 1991:156-162; Youngner et al., 1989: 2205; Youngner, 1992:2159-2161).

> On the other hand, while the [organ] donors are legally dead, they are members of a new class of dead patients about whom there is an even greater degree of discomfort...health professionals regularly use the term "braindead" to describe such patients, but only refer to them as "dead" when the ventilator is turned off after the organs have been removed. The latter time is regularly the one noted on death certificates. A recent study demonstrated that many health professionals are confused about their status; many do not really believe they are dead (Youngner, 1989).

(d) The dead body does not show the signs that has been traditionally associated with death. Or it does not appears altogether dead. This has also been reported as a source of normative and cognitive distress, both for health care personnel (Irwin, 1986; Sanner, 1991:163; Wolf, 1990:1019); and relatives (Irwin, 1986; Savaria et al., 1990:316-317):[132]

> These individuals do not appear dead, and they are treated in many ways as if they were alive in order to maintain the viability of organs for transplantation. Even those who understand and accept the concept of brain-death may find it difficult to ignore the signs of life they see. In the event of cardiopulmonary arrest, resuscitation may even be performed on a patient that has been declared dead (Irwin, 1986).

(e) The maintenance of these bodies (braindead donors) requires active monitoring and aggressive medication (e.g. cardiopulmonary resuscitation). Since these procedures are basically similar to the maintenance of patients in deep coma, the confusion experienced by relatives and the distress even among nursing personnel is increased (Youngner, 1966):

> Operating room [OR] personnel - nurses, were uncomfortable with the removal of life support in the OR, where usually every measure is taken to prevent death. They felt that strict supervision was necessary to prevent inappropriate removal of support and to ensure that support be removed humanely and without performing active euthanasia" (De Vita et al., 1993).

In sum, this technological development affects central concepts, values, norms and even rituals associated with dying and organ extraction within hospital settings.

The Living Body, the Braindead Body and the Corpse

The development of biological and medical knowledge has led to a conception of death as a process, characterised by more or less recognisable stages with diffuse boundaries. In this sense it is possible to talk about a functional death, a cellular death, etc. (Thomas, 1975). But death is also a *social process* conceptualised as the progressive ceasing of social functions (such as producing and consuming for instance).

The death of an individual – a biological as well as a social process – can be conceptualised as a process of progressive depersonalisation (as synonymous to dehumanisation) of the dead. This process is social since is characterised by corresponding social rules associated with each stage of "social death" (Sweeting, 1991). These social rules indicate what is the appropriate ritual treatment towards the body. The concepts of living/deceased/corpse are thus social categories, particular sets of relations (rule systems). The different concepts (terms) and rule systems entail different practices. Social behaviour towards deceased persons differs from that towards a patient in deep coma as opposed to a braindead "patient", or a corpse.

Consider the various ways of referring to the body in terms of the degree of humanness or "personality" it embodies. The "deceased" suggests a dead person, but she still has a name, relatives, testaments, property, and is, in a certain sense, sacred. The humanness of the corpse is only very abstract and general. The concept of "corpse" suggests a stage farther away from humanness, since the corpse has already lost most of its agency and as such enjoys less deference than that shown towards a deceased person. But even if the corpse is only a remains, it still may have a certain sacrality. The human cadaver, however, is socially decontextualised emphasising the more biological aspect of death. The depersonalisation or disconnection of the cadaver with human society is complete in that it is regarded as part of the "natural world" (such a concept *can be used for humans and animals alike)*. One can distinguish stages of de-personalisation also in medical practice. For instance, the autopsy is more upsetting to students than dissection, largely because the body is freshly dead and it is accompanied by personal information in the patient's medical record (Fox, 1979). It is much closer to everyday life than a cadaver ("smoked herring") in gross anatomy.

The process of social death of the dead is associated with rituals and ceremonies that mark the passage of the dead through stages of progressive depersonalisation. Each one of these different concepts has its proper place in corresponding contexts (as part of the social order). If the conceptual reference is altered and experienced as "wrong", uneasiness is experienced.[133] For example the use of a term such as "cadaver" in anatomy class is probably correct, but obviously less so when referring to somebody's dead relative in an intensive care unit.

Technically, in organ transplantation the process is similar, what is the patient as "person" in one extreme of a "personhood" scale ends as "biological material" in the other end (organs for transplantation with no connection to the personal characteristics of the dead donor).[134] However, in the case of the braindead donor, the passage of the dead person through these stages of progressive depersonalisation appear to be cognitively altered. In brain-death and organ harvesting, the characteristics of each stage of death and the corresponding social rules become blurred. This explains the ambiguous language and the multiplicity of terms (concepts) used in the literature to describe this category of deceased such as *"donor; organ donor; braindead patient; deceased; dead body"*:[135]

Confusion about the real status of potential donors (i.e. whether they are dead or alive) contributes to the emotional discomfort of those who must manage them in the intensive care unit or the operating room, e.g. the discomfort often felt by operating room personnel when the ventilator is turned off following organ retrieval surgery (Youngner et al., 1989).

Contemporary research shows that while there is a widespread acceptance of the whole brain criterion, there is also a confusion about its legal and clinical applications. Important reasons for this confusion among relatives and health care personnel alike are found in the similarity between the braindead and alive surgical patients in the operating room (OR) or patients in deep coma in the (neurological) intensive care unit (Youngner, 1996). Health professionals- have personal concepts of death that varied widely and are often confused and/or self-contradictory:

Not surprisingly the medical staff constantly used speech indicating that the patient was alive. "Our job was to keep the mother alive until the baby was born" one physician told me. A nurse said "We all *knew* that she was dead, but we *felt* she was alive". The patient's mother told a physician, "Every time I leave, I think she is going to finally die, and each time I return to the ICU she is still with us" (Youngner, 1996:47).

These transitions – or passages from patient, to braindead, to corpse (and finally cadaver) – are difficult, in part, because they entail danger and risk, namely treating an alive person as if she were dead, not distinguishing a dead person from the living, thinking and acting toward a dead person as if she were alive. Such confusion cannot be matters of innocent misunderstandings or mistakes. They can be the subject of professional, ethical, and legal judgements – and even evoke questions about one's rationality and humanity.

Clinical Versus Legal Categorisation: Conflicting Orientations and Rule Systems

At least two categorisations about death have been developed and applied in the course of the technological developments discussed earlier: one is legal categorisation, dichotomous and antinomic; the other is a clinical categorisation ultimately based on the notion of death as a process. The observable confusion and distress concerning the praxis of the maintenance of braindead for purposes of organ donation can be understood, in part, as the result of the two categorisations operating simultaneously. As Atkins (1992) suggests:

> The ambiguity inherent in organ transplantation is evidenced when we consider that we are being asked to accept a series of contradictions. Firstly, we are required to believe that the donor, on life support, is neither dead or alive, but both dead and alive. The organs are living but the person is dead. We must make a distinction between the body and the person. This fragmentation is arguably unfair since we can have no concept of a person which does not essentially involve the existence of a body (Atkins, 1992).

Legal categorisation defines a basic status of "living" or "dead". This classification is dichotomous and antinomic, in other words fine distinctions for example "dying" are excluded for legal purposes. This means that a dying individual is in principle entitled to the same rights as any other citizen. At the clinical level, however, distinctions such as *living/dead/ dead-dead* (Youngner, 1992); *living/braindead/dead* (Youngner, 1990), *living/dying/dead; living/living-dead/dead* (Wolf, 1990) are found.

While the introduction of legal measures was an important instrument in the resolution of some the tensions and conflicts experienced by medical personnel involved in organ procurement (i.e. before brain-death criteria were introduced), it prompted at the same time unintended consequences for those involved in the diagnosis (ICU physicians), maintenance (ICU nurses) and technical support (anaesthesiology and other operation (OP) nurses), and for general understandings of death.[136]

The moment when an individual is dead can be fixed as a cross-section in one point of a death process. *Optimally it should be the same, legally, medically and socially,* so that it is one and the same in legal, medical and social senses (Danish Council of Ethics, 1989:27). As pointed out by the Danish Council of Ethics (1989:27):

> The interest legal-technically and for the sake of the law and order has, until now, primarily consisted of a demand for clarity and practical applicability, including controllability... The choice between various criteria is ultimately and predominantly a politico-culturally decided choice in which, inter alia, regard to the deceased and the relatives of the deceased, must be "weighted against" a more or less widespread demand for organs and so forth. The legal interest consists in describing the control problems which arise in . connection with possibly changed death criteria, the problems which might arise in respect to the traditional differentiation between a corpse and a living person as well as the problems which might arise in connection with (delimitation of) the use of persons whose brain function has ceased.

In sum:

(1) The distinction between living and dead is crucial in everyday life,

in law and in medicine.

(2) Particular techniques and technological developments have led to shifts in the boundaries between living and dead and, in particular, the divergence of legal, clinical and everyday distinctions. This is not just a problem of correct measurements, as indicated earlier (although there are different opinions about measurements and how to interpret them). The braindead do not appear dead in most instances, and they are not treated as simply dead either.

(3) The lack of correspondence or harmony between legal and clinical definitions (as well as everyday conceptions) results in ambiguity, confusion and stress for medical and nursing personnel. It is also a problem for the general public.

(4) The "ambiguous body" refers to the fact that the braindead body is an *intermediate bodily state* between the dead and the alive body, a state constructed through life-sustaining systems and largely in response to the demand for organs.[137] The transition from braindead (a dead but living body) to dead body (the "second death") occurs when blood circulation and respiratory functions cease (for example when life-sustaining devices are intentionally turned off in the operating theatre). Moreover, one can discern as well the role in law in mediating between the medical world and the common-sensical or everyday world of citizens. This serves to maintain the legitimacy of medical institutions and personnel dealing with the complexity and ambiguity of brain-death and organ procurement situations. The law accomplishes this in part by defining what actions are permitted and which forbidden, thus creating a sense – a social fact – that an area of great danger and risk is regulated by explicit rules determined by agents with no special interest in the area.

The construction of an intermediate bodily state, the braindead, between the living and the corpse, is an unintended consequence of the widespread use of intensive care technologies, together with the growing demand for the use of human tissue and organs, and consequently the changes in traditional death criteria. But these developments entail the loss of correspondence between legal, clinical and everyday conceptions of living bodies.

Conclusion: Medical Technological Innovation and Destabilisation of Established Clinical Discourses and Rituals

The destabilisation produced by the introduction of formal-legal and clinical classifications regarding the braindead is of systematic and enduring character. Conventional strategies and practices tend to fail. The stage is set for organisational, legal, and ethical challenges and innovations. New discourses, institutional arrangements and rituals emerge. But the process of learning, normalisation and achievement of a new stabilisation is often a slow one. The specialised literature as well as my interviews suggest a series of sociopsychological problems among both relatives and personnel related to the care and maintenance of the braindead, problems characterised by ambiguity and dissonance. As pointed out earlier, the introduction of procedures to keep a dead patient functioning, in a sense "alive-like", until the organs can be removed leads to ambiguous and dissonant situations (Chapter 7). Also the continuous pressures to act more efficiently and to minimise "delays" makes timing and the arrangements of the organ procurement take precedence over the feelings of the next-of-kin.

The introduction of new conceptions as well as techniques and technologies lead to new classifications, e.g. in this case brain-death. While the law distinguishes simply between alive and dead defined as brain-death, clinical practices distinguish between the braindead and the finally dead (the "dead-dead") (see previous section). Clinical practice (intensive care units) makes such distinctions since it works with a type of dead (the braindead) who are in a state that is clearly distinguishable from the non-heart-beating dead-dead (which are dealt with in entirely different ways, for example sent to the morgue of the hospital, cremated, etc.).

The intermediate or transitional states, such as that of brain-death in clinical practice, are often ambiguous or liminal (the ambiguous grey zone between classifications as defined in Turner's (1969) terms). It is not surprising that actors experienced ambiguity and a sense of risk or threat (Gennep, 1977). The intermediate state disturbs established rituals and discourses for dealing with the dead, even among experienced medical personnel.

As discussed in Chapter 8, there are numerous accounts of rituals performed by nurses and physicians in the hospital (Chapman, 1983; Elks, 1996), for example in relation to the deceased (Wolf, 1988, 1989), to stillborn and dead infants (Andersson Wretmark, 1994). Rituals and ritualised behaviour in health care help to: (a) order experiences in critical situations, contributing to a sense of security and control over the situation; (b) reaffirm meaning(s) in unclear situations; (c) strengthen community or professional ties when collectively performed. Many established rituals for dealing with the dying and the dead are disrupted by the maintenance and use of braindead donors and become a source of distress for many nurses.

In general, the problems of ambiguity and dissonance are particularly prominent under conditions of social or socio-technical change, for instance when new techniques and technologies are introduced that affect important normative or sensitive areas of social life. The technological developments relating to brain-death and organ transplantation confront the involved actors with new types of problems: experiences of ambiguity and dissonance arising in the context of modifying the boundaries between life and death and affecting, for example, nursing practices including rituals and "proper ways" of treating the dead.

For such cases, the established routines, criteria for judgement, procedures, etc. no longer lead to the minimisation of ambiguity and the reduction of dissonance, but rather to their intensification. *Of particular importance is the way in which innovations in techniques and technologies may not only alter established procedures and information and accounting systems but also disrupt discourses and rituals that earlier had contributed to effectively stabilising judgements concerning life or death questions.* That is, actors experience new types of ambiguities and dissonance – or old ones which can no longer be readily or systematically resolved or minimised through established organisational means (discussed in Chapter 7 and 8).

7 Dissonance in the Hospital

Introduction[138]

The hospital, medical and nursing literature (for example, *Transplantation Proceedings*, *Journal of Advanced Nursing*, *New Journal of Medicine*, *Journal of the American Medical Association* and *The Kennedy Institute of Ethics Journal*, among others) reports tensions, anxieties and frequent difficulties among personnel dealing with organ donation and braindead patients. My own interviews and hospital observations in Sweden have also brought to light such problems. Often the explanations of such stress among health care personnel have been psychological, even existential, a type of human anguish in the face of death (Sanner, 1991),[139] an "irrational" or "over-emotional" behaviour. More general explanations attribute the problems to inadequate or insufficient socialisation and to general states of anxiety or anguish in difficult medical settings. Particularly noteworthy is that these problems have been reported in several different countries practising organ transplantation and dealing with braindead patients. In the course of my research, I discovered patterns in the cognitive and emotional problems arising in these medical settings. The following analysis – and illustrations – primarily address the situation of medical personnel, and collaterally that of next-of-kin. The actors involved occupy different positions or roles in the hospital context (physicians, nurses and relatives). The study points up also some aspects of the sociological significance of death and dying. In the human confrontation with death, one of the most marginal situations to taken-for-granted everyday reality, the transcendental potency of symbolic universes manifests itself most clearly (Berger and Luckman, 1967:119).

Several researchers (Chan, 1991; Keatings, 1990; Machado, 1996; Youngner et al., 1988, 1989a, 1989b) have suggested that these problems are basically the result of a rupture or destabilisation of cognitive and emotional frames (Goffman (1974) speaks generally about the "vulnerability of perceptual frames"). Cognitive dissonance theory or, more generally, cognitive balance theories are a useful point of departure to analyse and explain these problems. In the following sections, I summarise the classical psychological theory, before going on to outline an organisational theory. The latter is used to identify patterns of cognitive imbalance and to explain why such imbalance is problematic in the medical situations under study. The theory combines cognitive concepts (frames, cognitions, beliefs, judgements, dissonance, etc.) with organisational (positions, roles, relations, authority, social order) and cultural concepts (shared or collective representations, judgements frames, rituals, discourses).

Psychological Theories of Cognitive Balance and Dissonance

Classical psychological cognitive balance theories (Abelson et al., 1968; Aronson, 1995; Brehm and Cohen, 1962; Festinger, 1957; Heider, 1858; Zajonc, 1968a, 1968b; among others) deal largely with individual experiences of imbalance and the stabilising responses to imbalance or dissonance.[140] Cognitions are defined as items of belief, knowledge, and judgement that a person may hold or experience at a given time – knowledge, belief, or judgement about oneself, one's environment or one's behaviour. An action taken is experienced or cognised, and enters into complex cognitive processes. Cognitions can be *consonant* (compatible), *dissonant* (contradictory) or *irrelevant* to each other. The association between cognitions has a psychological rather than logical character (cultural premises, pressures to be logical, behavioural commitment, past experience, etc.). Schematically, the major propositions of the theory according to Zajonc (1968a, 1968b) are: (1) Cognitive dissonance is an aversive state; (2) the individual will attempt to reduce, eliminate or avoid events that produce or increase cognitive dissonance; (3) the severity or the intensity of the cognitive dissonance varies with the importance, and the relative number, of cognitions standing in dissonant relation to one another; (4) cognitive dissonance can be reduced or eliminated by adding new cognitions or by changing existing ones; (5) the new cognitions may throw added weight to one side, decreasing the proportion of cognitions which are dissonant; (6) the added cognitions may change the importance of the cognitive elements that are in dissonant relation with one another; (7) cognitions may change and become less important or less contradictory with others; (8) these processes may foster other behaviours which have cognitive consequences favouring consonance, such as seeking new information. Three major mechanisms of reducing dissonance postulated are: (a) information selectivity, (b) reinterpretation, and (c) redefinition of the situation.[141]

Festinger and others (Festinger, 1957; also Festinger and Carlsmith, 1959; Festinger et al., 1956; Aronson, 1968, 1969, 1995, among many others) formulated the theory of *cognitive dissonance in terms of individual reactions to dissonant or incongruent cognitions.*[142] Whenever there is a concern with groups (e.g. in Festinger et al. (1956)), one simply aggregates the cognitive experiences and responses of individuals.

An Organisational Theory

My point of departure is to stress the organisational basis of key cognitive processes and the role of such processes in the construction and maintenance of the social order of hospital units. In this perspective, the generation of cognitive imbalance – as well as resolution processes – are embedded in an organisational structure: in particular, an organisation's division of function and labour, its distribution of responsibility and authority, its institutionalised roles, discourses and rituals. Thus, I transform what has largely been a social psychological approach into an organisational theory, grounding cognitive balance – and balancing processes – in the organisational or institutional contexts where these phenomena occur.

The *Organisational Theory of Cognitive Balance* (*hereafter OTC*) specifies and analyses the ways in which such cognitive processes operate in organisational contexts and through organisational mechanisms. The hospital is viewed as a particular social order, in which key groups of actors, physicians and nurses utilise a particular perspective, a cognitive-normative or judgement frame (Burns, 1990; Burns et al., 1997; Goffman, 1974; Taylor, 1989). This frame serves not only as a common basis for organising perceptions, making judgements and decisions and for acting so as to shape and maintain a particular social order. But it also serves as a basis for self-definition and identity as well as definitions of authority, status, and prestige relations.

Physicians, for example, are responsible and accountable for making correct distinctions or judgements that are intended to save a patient's life or to relieve a patient's suffering; they also make judgements about what is the prognosis for a patient, or the usefulness of a dying patient's organs for transplantation, or the question of whether a patient is alive, close to death, or dead. Such determinations are the basis for particular social acts, and further judgements. *The "correct" determination of whether or not a patient is "dead" or "alive"*[143] – *and the "proper" action(s) to take on the basis of such judgements – has professional, legal, moral, and social implications.* This is of particular significance to physicians, medical personnel, and hospital administrators since they are accountable for this judgement and actions taken on the basis of such a judgement. Clearly, one acts differently, has different responsibilities, obligations, rights toward a living person than toward a dead person. The same act in the two situations may be in one case permissible or even required, and in the other wrongful or even criminal. For example, the act of turning off the ventilator such that the patient stops breathing may, depending on contextual factors and conditions, be defined or interpreted as "homicide", "helping the patient to die", "letting the patient die" (that is, doing nothing to save the patient, or "allowing nature take her course"); or dealing properly with patients defined as braindead. If a patient is judged by a physician to be "dead", according to brain-death criteria, the removal of a life-support system is neither an illegal nor an unethical act.

Those who have the responsibility for making correct judgements interact with one another within a socially defined order, the hospital administrative and professional order. This is constituted and regulated by more or less shared systems of rules and procedures for orienting, categorising, evaluating, judging and acting in the situation (Burns and Flam, 1987). That is, the judgements concerning life and death are made within a particular organisational and cognitive framework according to certain judgement criteria, procedures, and discourses.

The professionals in the hospital setting, in particular physicians and nurses, act on the basis of particular beliefs, cognitions, and judgements. They commit themselves cognitively but also in concrete actions and allocation of resources. As already indicated, much is at stake here: legally, professionally, and morally. The cognitive, emotional, and action commitment sets the stage for the experience of cognitive disturbance and imbalance. *This is not just a factual problem but a problem of legal and moral responsibility as well as professional status and prestige.*[144] In this type of situation, the professional actors are highly motivated to establish a clear distinction or boundary between states or types of "situation", for instance between different types of illness or different stages of "life" and "death".[145]

In constructing and maintaining the hospital order, key professional actors share, then, certain definitions: a "definition of reality", "social facts", to which participating actors orient and take into account in framing their conceptions, their judgements, and actions. Thus, there is a solid basis for knowing which rules and roles apply, which classification schemes to use, which frames of meaning and interpretations are valid or legitimate. Actors are empowered with the capacity to co-ordinate activities, and to give accounts, and to critically reflect on what is happening. There is some degree – but not complete – "closure" with respect to extraneous or incongruous pieces of information, data, and communications.

The theory consists of two fundamental principles:

I. *Cognitive imbalance is generated through the experience of events, actions, and communications that contradict shared judgement frames or particular cognitive and behavioural commitments made in the professional and organisational context of a hospital.* Cognitive imbalance according to OTC is generated within organisations (and resolved, if and when resolution is accomplished) in the context of commitments to organisationally key beliefs, judgements, and actions which are contradicted by events or communications, or other data. Only a small subset of all the diverse imbalance experiences are considered collectively relevant, and responded to with collectively activated or collectively recognised means.[146] Salient cognitions relate to, symbolise, or derive from aspects of the hospital order, giving the organisation its identity, its core values and norms, and its key authority, status and role relationships: namely, (1) values in medical contexts such as the sacrality of life and orientation to the welfare of patients; (2) norms directing members to do their utmost to save lives, to care properly for patients, to perform in competent or professional ways; (3) shared judgement frames based to a considerable degree on medical knowledge and techniques; (4) organisational authority and status relationships which are grounded in certification and demonstration of medical competence (rather than legal correctness, business success, or coercion). These components of the social order are highly salient features for *common* experiences of cognitive imbalance and the utilisation of established balancing mechanisms within an organisation. At least this is the case for actors in positions of major responsibility and authority such as physicians and leading nurses.

The professionals occupying key positions of authority and status are not only major representatives and carriers of hospital order but are those expected – and expecting themselves – to engage in and confront events, actions, and communications that are problematic for the order. In their leading positions and roles in the hospital organisation they represent and act in terms of – and defend – a particular judgement frame. That is, given their positions in the order, they are *committed* to particular cognitive states and related judgements, decisions, and actions concerning critical, possibly life or death, matters. Imbalance arises because a cognition to which actors are committed – or commit themselves in the course of their ongoing activities – is contradicted by actual experience, communications from others, or other incoming information. Such contradiction arises because the actors are compelled to act but lack full control over what happens and over relevant information flows. There is a significant degree of uncontrollability and unpredictability (see below).[147]

Often there are strong emotional reactions to dissonant experiences: professional members may react with anger, deep embarrassment, sense of profound failure and distress, etc. The reaction to some challenges is "righteous anger", for which members have the moral right – and even duty – to react, to chastise, and to punish (Collins, 1988). Burke (1991) sees such social distress arising from disruption or interruption of one's sense of self, a self which is continually salient and being generated; that is, the identity process is affected by the evaluations, communications, and actions of others – as well as those of members of the profession and organisation itself. The diffuse anxiety this produces is a major force of motivation (and relates to Giddens' notion that the control of diffuse anxiety is the most generalised motivational origin of human conduct (Giddens, 1984:154)). In order to deal with this, people make use of various institutionalised strategies (as outlined below). Such strategies, may, however, never reach the conscious awareness of the participants even in the case of an organisation dominated by highly educated and knowledgeable professionals.

II. *Organisationally significant instances of cognitive imbalance and dissonance are resolved through institutionalised means or strategies, above all particular organisational arrangements, rituals and discourses.* These are institutionalised means to reduce imbalance or dissonance: that is, they entail particular means of information selectivity, re-interpretation of data and information, and re-definition of the saliency or relevancy of dissonant information. The resolution or reduction problematique in such cases is not left to individuals, but is dealt with in collectively established and legitimate ways. Ritual and discourse are both communicative means to convey meaning, to deal with contradiction and dissonance, and to maintain normative order and cognitive solidarity (Acquili et al., 1979; Burns and Laughlin, 1979; Douglas, 1987).

For instance, through organisational procedures, rituals, and discourses, a dissonant cognition may be blocked or altered; or the importance of one cognition may be decreased to the advantage of another; or a justification may be made for ignoring or emphasising one cognition in relation to another. Selectivity can occur through discourses stressing, for instance, technical data and medical scientific concepts and excluding other types of information as "irrelevant". Information may be selected (or conversely, excluded) so as to stabilise particular cognitions or judgements, for instance that a patient is braindead (although appearing in some ways to be alive). Or discourses may operate to reinterpret data in such a way as to provide a sense of consonance or balance by redefining a cognition or experience as irrelevant, and, therefore, a condition or situation of non-responsibility or non-commitment. In such a way, the imbalanced state is re-framed or re-structured, and balance is restored. Moreover, the process contributes to the *shared* experience of cognitive stability.[148] Participating actors communicate or express their commitment and loyalty to the hospital order through particular rituals and discourses, among other things, dealing with disturbances or challenges to the order from insiders as well as outsiders. A sense of shared meanings and right and proper order are maintained.

In general, many organisational arrangements and practices including rituals and special discourses answer to immediate organisational or professional ends. For instance, they do not make health care more efficient or better. Rather, they operate to defend the normative order and cognitive solidarity against imbalance, dissonance or contradiction, and a sense of disorder.

Not all – possibly not even most – experiences of cognitive imbalance or dissonance are disturbing or distressful. People are tolerant of a wide variety of inconsistencies and contradictions (Aronson, 1992; Billig et al., 1988). Three conditions make for hospital or clinical situations where professionals experience contradiction and cognitive imbalance as problematic and distressful:

a) Collective identity and commitment. Hospitals are a type of organisation, where physicians and nurses,[149] core professional groups, embody and apply a particular judgement or cognitive-normative frame (Burns et al., 1997). Such a frame is a contextualised social construction for making reality judgements, value judgements, and problem-solving and action judgements in particular socially defined contexts. The frame consists of collective representations, definitions of reality, and relevant values, norms, and other rules. The collective representations and definitions are types of shared cognitive maps used by actors in orienting themselves and determining their actions as well as in interpreting ongoing activities in the hospital.[150] They are also important in the giving and asking of accounts of professional activities. Situationally relevant rules, including norms and values, orient the actors in their positions and roles, regarding what they should do, how they should do it, what are the conditions for doing it, and what are "right and proper" or "good" as opposed to "bad" actions in the context(s) in which they operate. Thus, the established judgement frame is the basis of a certain degree of inter-subjectivity, common judgements, mutual understandings, and, in general, a collective capacity to reflect upon and construct reality together (Burns and Engdahl, 1998).

The professionals embodying and representing the shared judgement frame are already committed – and commit themselves in the course of making judgements and taking actions in their work – to particular definitions of reality and particular beliefs, judgements, and actions (and the principles underlying these). At the core of the judgement frame is a conception of collective as well as individual professional selves – that is, *identities* – for orientating toward and interacting with others. A profession's collective self and the individual professional selves are thus bound up with a particular *cognitive field* (Burns and Engdahl, 1998). A key component in the cognitive field is a definition of reality – a social fact – that the professionals are genuinely trustworthy in at least two senses: (1) physicians as well as nurses have technical expertise; their medical practices are understood or defined as "scientific"; (2) the judgement(s) and actions of physicians and nurses are ethically right and proper – they care about patients and try to do their best in treating them. Members react when components of their cognitive field are contradicted or challenged.

Burke and Reitzes (1991) stress identity or self-conception as a major source of motivation for action, particularly action seen as relevant or expressive for the realisation of identity. Conversely, an actor is predisposed to avoid acting – and being defined – in ways contradicting or inconsistent with her self-conception or identity. While a concern with particular "choices" or decisions is of major interest, often more important are *commitments* to action, judgement, or statement – which turn out, however, to result in contradictions with self-conception or cognitive elements closely connected with it. A significant public performance or outcome, a *fait accompli*, however, which contradicts identity or closely associated cognitions sets the stage for experiences of dissonance, distress, and the activation of stabilising mechanisms.

b) Responsibility and demand for commitment to action. Problematic or significant cognitive imbalance or dissonance arises in connection with a collective conception or definition of the *social order of the organisation*, and its core, the authoritative professions of physicians and nurses. A participant, because of her position or role, feels connected to, "responsible for", or "engaged" in the particular cognition, belief, or decision, or action. She is motivated to orient to and deal with situations or information that contradict, challenge, threaten, destabilise or confuse key aspects of the organisational order, or an actor's particular position, her authority and status in it (or both). Major relevant aspects of the order are organisational and professional self-conceptions, core values and norms, key authority and status relations, and the shared judgement frame as well as the particular cognitions, decisions, and actions derived from or generated within that order. In a word, the cognitive imbalance, dissonance, or contradiction is professionally or organisationally salient or relevant.

Organisationally relevant situations for possible cognitive imbalance arise whenever core professionals, occupying defined organisational positions and playing particular roles, are responsible for the situation and must commit themselves to action (including commitments to particular judgements, decisions, and initiatives). These actors are accountable for their decisions and actions and, at the same time, must commit themselves in a significant matter, for example in assessing whether or not a person has a particular illness and should be treated in specific ways, or in reacting to the fact that a person is dying, or in determining whether a patient is alive or dead. Failure to make proper determinations means that one may act improperly or illegally in dealing with a patient. For example, one might inadvertently commit or serve as an accessory to a homicide by attending/medicating/treating a living person as dead. On the other hand, treating a dead person as living – a type of problem arising in connection with using life support systems to maintain the braindead prior to organ harvesting – is also highly problematic. There are professional, administrative, legal, and social reasons for this, as we shall see. In sum, organisationally and professionally *salient* experiences of cognitive imbalance arise in connection with experiences which contradict characteristic or core elements of the hospital's social and cognitive order to which the professionals are committed and for which they feel responsible.

c) Absence of complete control in relevant situations. Instances of cognitive imbalance arise because the actors responsible for making decisions and commitments to action lack complete control over what happens. Nonetheless, they are responsible. In many decision and action situations there is some degree of uncertainty, uncontrollability, and unpredictability. Events occur, experiences and data are generated, which contradict the cognitive orientation (or judgements and actions based on it), thus setting the stage for experiences of cognitive imbalance or dissonance. The hospital order, while highly institutionalised, is vulnerable in a number of ways to challenges, confrontations, communications, experiences, etc. that confuse, threaten, challenge, or destabilise professional self-conceptions as well as conceptions of the hospital as a professional organisation. Thus, individuals and groups in the hospital setting are particularly sensitive toward, and respond to, communications from others that question key assumptions and meanings of the hospital order. In particular, events, communications, judgements, and specific performances may contradict the belief or cognition that medical personnel and organisations genuinely care about patients, try to save lives, relieve discomfort and pain, and accomplish this through the systematic application of scientific-medical expertise and techniques. A highly sensitive area for the experience of cognitive imbalance relates to issues of hospital authority, power, and status relationships. These are grounded and legitimised not only on the basis of a manifest concern for patients but on the systematic application of medical and scientific knowledge and techniques. Events, experiences, or communications that indicate, or might be interpreted as indicating, incompetence in dealing with, or obvious disregard for, the welfare of, patients tend to generate cognitive dissonance. A related, highly salient area of collective concern and response relates to contradictory messages or challenges with respect to medical and scientific definitions and interpretations of reality.

Cognitive inconsistencies and imbalance occur when performances, events, communications, and developments, on the one hand, clash with definitions, beliefs, judgements, intended or expected actions and outcomes, on the other. In part, this occurs because the former are never fully under hospital or professional control, or so orderly or unproblematic that they "fit" or are perfectly congruent. Some immediate corrections may be possible to make, but often these are a *fait accompli*, the result of commitments or statements made, actual performances carried out, or more or less objective outcomes. The hospital, the core professions, their legitimacy, their authority, status, or prestige are at stake: they may be challenged or appear in a bad light, or make for professional embarrassment or shame, unless properly and effectively addressed, for example through particular discourses and rituals.

The OTC perspective on cognitive imbalance and resolution can be summarised as follows:

Figure 9. Cognitive imbalance and resolution processes

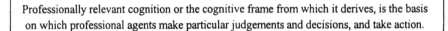

Professionally relevant cognition or the cognitive frame from which it derives, is the basis on which professional agents make particular judgements and decisions, and take action.

Information, experience, or data obtained within the organisational context lead to one or more cognitions that contradict the original cognition, judgement, or action.

Experience of cognitive imbalance or dissonance (typically varying by position and role in the organisation).

Organisational discourses, rituals and other devices reduce or eliminate imbalance (these ways possibly varying by position and role in the organisation).

Professionals occupy positions within a hospital organisation – and play particular roles – which entail commitments to an established judgement frame as well as derived commitments to particular beliefs, situational cognitions, judgements and actions. In our study here, physicians and nurses – the core professional groups in hospital settings – embody collective self-conceptions and particular judgement frames.[151] A judgement frame is part of – is closely connected to – professional self-conception or identity. It consists of collective representations and classification schemes, particular beliefs, norms and values, and conceptions or definitions of role, authority and status relationships (all of these components will be specified and discussed more fully in the following sections). Professional identities commit their members to – holds them responsible for – key cognitive and normative components of the judgement frame (this includes cognitions, judgements, and actions derived from or closely connected with applications of the frame). Experiences, communications, or other forms of data, which contradict or are incongruent with one or more such components or their derivatives cause distress and evoke balancing processes. Professional actors in the hospital experience salient contradiction and imbalance and activate and participate in institutionalised balancing processes. Through particular organisational and professional rituals and discourses, hospital professionals define their commitment to and reinforcement of professional identity or selfhood; they also express loyalty and commitment to particular values and norms, particular roles, authority and status relations. Throughout this and the following chapter, OTC explores *the dynamic interlinkage between professional identity and normative commitments, cognitive processes, and ritualistic and emotional order and solidarity.* These factors are all part and parcel of the social construction of the hospital order.

Cognitive Imbalance vis-à-vis Brain Death and Organ Retrieval

Critical Situations: High-Tech Death

The application of criteria of irreversible brain failure in defining death builds on advanced technology and specialised knowledge. This contrasts significantly with "common sense" notions of death.[152] As a result, brain death is often a difficult notion for many people to comprehend. The dividing line between a patient in deep coma and a "patient" defined as braindead is not clear-cut, and to identify an individual in this condition as dead by irreversible brain failure is not within the competence of non-professionals, but only of trained physicians. However, a braindead patient sustained by a respirator does not exhibit obvious differences from a living but comatose patient.[153] The signs that configure the status of brain death in a patient are assessed by a clinical examination, and in certain circumstances also by additional tests to assess the viability of the brain.[154] It is also understandable that the confusion regarding brain death experienced by relatives of the deceased can be augmented when, for purposes of maintaining the organs viable for transplantation, the deceased is actively monitored and medicated by the personnel of an intensive care unit. The determination of death according to brain-death criteria has been subject to controversies inside and outside the medical profession (Horton and Horton, 1991:1048; De Vita and Snyder, 1993:136; De Vita, Snyder and Gränvik, 1993:113-129; Veatch, 1993; Brante and Hallberg, 1989).

There is a metaphoric but also potential cognitive gap between the notion of a more "straightforward" death, supposedly easier for everybody to identify by generic signs (prolonged unresponsiveness, absence of respiration and heart beat, pallor, and coldness) and the more "indirect" conception of irreversible brain failure, where the (tangible) signs of death are not revealed immediately and can only be discerned by a professional using proper techniques and equipment.[155] Notwithstanding, brain death can present difficulties even for medical and nursing personnel in intensive and emergency wards who are responsible for the viability and maintenance of a deceased person for purposes of organ procurement.

In situations of particular interest here, the actor(s) responsible (usually together with her/their "colleagues") have committed themselves and others to a particular belief or judgement and acted on the basis of it. Afterwards, contradictory information may be obtained that gives rise to quandaries about the appropriateness of the action, even if it does not directly challenge the correctness of the judgement. That is, the situation may appear differently than initially believed or judged. A dissonance may arise between judgement (or belief) about a state of the world and an experience of the actual situation.[156] Or it may arise between what one does (or did) and what one should do (or should have done). In part, *this implies lack of total control over the situation or over the data generated.*

The notion that someone may appear dead but may be alive, is an old one, and the stuff of numerous stories (fictional as well as real). With the development of high-tech death, the possibilities of appearing alive, but defined as dead, according to brain-death criteria have increased dramatically. Cognitive imbalance may be generated in such situations in that a patient is defined or believed to be dead but personnel (as well as next-of-kin) experience signs incompatible with this cognition, and the medical actions based on it, such as removing organs. For instance, a braindead patient may jerk or move as a result of spinal reflexes. This challenges beliefs about the responses of a properly dead person.

Reports of hospital personnel experiencing cognitive and emotional disturbances and stress in connection with brain-death situations are common (Chan, 1992; Keatings, 1990; Youngner et al., 1988, 1989a, 1989b, 1992; among others), and often concern the fact that there are discrepancies and uncertainties in connection with the patient's status. Many nurses do not consistently experience braindead patients as truly dead, for instance those whose organs are to be extracted (Wolf, 1990). Irwin (1986:306) observes:

> These individuals do not appear dead, and they are treated in many ways as if they were alive in order to maintain the viability of organs for transplantation. Even those who understand and accept the concept of brain death may find it difficult to ignore the signs of life they see. In the event of cardiopulmonary arrest, resuscitation may even be performed on a patient that has been declared dead.

Youngner et al. (1989:2205) also points out that many professionals are confused about braindead patients (and the status of the donor). The discomfort of the physicians and nurses who work with these patients, especially in the operating room, has been described extensively in the literature (Youngner, 1988:439). Arnold and Youngner (1993:267) report that almost a third of the physicians and nurses in their studies did not perceive such patients as dead at all but accepted treating them as dead because they were irreparably damaged or death was imminent (see also Tomlinson:1990).

The relatives of braindead patients also express difficulties in integrating the physical signs with the report from the physician or nurse that their relative is dead.[157] Pelletier (1992) reports a number of factors that made it difficult for family members to accept the brain death diagnosis: the patients' show signs of viability, such as *breathing or a beating heart; or normal body functions such as warmth, perspiration, and hair growth.* Moreover, reports such as the following are common:

> They [the relatives] see that he [braindead] gets nourishment and diuretics through a tube, he sweats, urinates and they see the electroencephalograph connected. *It is difficult to associate it with death* (Sanner, 1991:159).

> Actually "parting" with the patient when he or she does not seem to be fully dead was thus a problem for many of the survivors. Usually this reluctance manifests itself in a delay in the decision process while the surviving family members come to terms with the alternatives. Although she did not go to this extreme, one mother admitted, *"You know, you have second thoughts too [such as] I could bring him home on one of those machines... I could take care of him"* (Fulton et al., 1977:356).

> One woman said – "[My husband's] mother couldn't get it through her head - she felt that as long as his heart was beating and he was breathing he was alive" (Fulton et al., 1977:354).

> One spouse remembered that his [her husband's] heart was pumping away when he was pronounced dead. "He appeared alive yet he [the physician] had just told me he was dead. How could I believe he was dead?" (Pelletier: 1992:93).

Given the experience of uncertainty around brain death, it is not surprising that many next-of-kin fear that their braindead relative suffers or will suffer during organ extraction (Youngner et al., 1990; Sanner, 1991; among others) These feelings follow, in part, from the physical signs of "life" in the deceased. As indicated above, this is a common concern expressed by relatives:

> Acts performed upon the cadaver immediately following death are commonly felt, emotionally, to be acts upon a still sentient individual, as I have experienced when requesting permission for autopsy: *"Oh, doctor, hasn't he suffered enough already?"* (Emson, 1987:125).

> Fear of mutilation and suffering was frequently verbalised, although relatives could barely define the nature and cause of the fear (Fernandez et al., 1991:1800).

In general, the braindead conception, technologies, and experiences appear to make the acceptance of death by next-of-kin more difficult. Denial of death is often present, especially when the family can observe the breathing movements (maintained by the respirator) (Fernandez et al.,1991).

Organisational Roles and Patterns of Cognitive Imbalance

A key principle in our conception of cognitive imbalance generated and patterned by the organisational structure is that major types of imbalance relate to the identity of the organisation, its core values and norms, its key professionals. The core values in medical settings consist of saving lives, caring for patients, relieving discomfort and pain through the application of scientific-medical knowledge and technologies. Different medical personnel will tend to comprehend and evaluate any given situation as a function of their positions and roles in the organisation. They have (a) varying responsibilities, powers, and decision-making conditions; (b) different training, different orientations and concerns such that they deal with different types of information; and (c) none of them have access to all the information. Consequently, *the patterns of experiencing and resolving cognitive imbalance are likely to vary among actors and groups of actors in the organisation.* In other words, the organisational division of function and labour makes for positional differences in imbalance experiences and in available balancing mechanisms. *Actors in their different positions or roles experience different degrees and even types of imbalance. Likewise, the ways of dealing with different dissonances will tend to vary among actors playing different roles.*[158] In particular, they will have available and utilise diverse organisational and professional discourses and rituals in the cognitive balancing processes. Of interest here are actors occupying different positions or playing different roles in hospital settings with respect to death and dying as well as questions of organ removal, specifically: (1) attending or responsible physicians, (2) nurses, (3) next-of-kin.

Reports in the hospital and professional literature indicate dissonance experiences for all three groups; our own empirical investigations lend support to these reports. Below we briefly examine the distinct forms of cognitive imbalance and balancing processes in the three groups:

(1) The physician: agency and responsibility in defining situations and determining commitment to action. Attending physicians are responsible and have authority in the hospital setting to determine if a patient is "dying", or dead. Nonetheless, this is not a simple medical matter where the attending physician is a sovereign. First, judgements may be reviewed and held accountable by other physicians (adhering, however, to more or less the same professional frame for making such judgements, the same methods and procedures). Second, and perhaps more significantly, the physician has to take into account legal (as well as ethical) considerations, the fact that legally death is understood as a moment or event in time. Thus, there are different judgement frames and rules which may come into conflict and *set the stage for dissonance: for instance, the medical/scientific frame coming into opposition with the legal one.*

(2) The nurses: engagement with limited agency (and subordinate knowledge). Nurses are typically not in a position to make the judgement or commitment (corresponding to the empowerment and responsibility of physicians). They are accessories to the physicians, and implement decisions. They observe many of the consequences of decisions or obtain information relevant to decisions and commitments. Nurses experience organisationally generated imbalance when they observe conditions or obtain data that do not fit with the physicians' authoritative definition of reality and action commitments: a braindead patient reacts in ways that appear living, or the braindead individual is maintained by means of life-support. However, even if the nursing personnel have less to say about radical procedures (particularly in intensive care units, where the activities have a highly technical character), by virtue of their particular professional training they notice and manage information that differs from the information to which physicians orient.

(3)   The next-of-kin: outsiders facing the definitions provided by authorities. Next-of-kin are typically ignorant of procedures, for example intensive care units. They have limited insight and access to medical data and the medical definitions of the situation. They seldom understand the legal implications, either. Some of what they are told or are led to understand does not necessarily fit with what they believe, or have thought or known. They may have doubts or suspicions – they may even refuse to believe or try to deny the information that, for example, their relative is dead. But ultimately they are dependent on and must rely on medical authority to interpret and define the situation.

In all of these cases, the various actors find themselves in situations where *their reality frames are vulnerable* (Goffman, 1974), *but where their differing frames are vulnerable in different ways*. The source of vulnerability for the physician and his medical conception is his professional accountability as well as legal responsibility (that is, accountability even outside of the medical system). Intensive and emergency care nurses usually understand the concept of brain-death. Also, the physician's authority to determine if a patient is living, dying or dead (in other words, to define the reality of the situation) is decisive. However, they may find some of the "dead" patients they deal with as problematic because they do not look dead enough. In cases where patient organs will be utilised for organ transplantation they have to be "maintained and monitored" by nursing personnel until organ harvesting can be carried out. (The bodies have to be heavily medicated in order to maintain a good circulation of blood in the organs, sufficient production of urine, level of temperature, etc.; also these "patients" receive cardio-pulmonary resuscitation if the heart should fail). In short, in a number of different ways, the nursing personnel of the ICUs must provide support to these deceased "as if they are alive". Finally, next-of-kin must rely on physicians and nurses to tell them the status of their sick, dying, or dead relatives. Still, they may not comprehend much of what is being said or determined, for example what is the nature of "brain death". Non-medical actors observe and express concern about dissonant data (for instance, their "braindead" relative appears to be in a "coma"). This, in many cases, may be explained away or dismissed by the medical authorities with whom they are in contact. But they are driven to seek explanation and certainty, not only about the status of their relative but about the right and proper actions to be taken under the circumstances. There are numerous reports in the medical literature about such problems and our own investigations corroborate the significance of these problems.

Implications of the Theory and Analytic Results

I. Being a member of a profession or a professional organisation such as a hospital means having a more or less common standpoint or frame for organising perception and determining judgement and action (for a general consideration of this conception, see Burns et al., 1997; Goffman, 1974; Machado and Burns, 1998; Taylor, 1989). The frame defines a professional standpoint or perspective: the conception of, or beliefs about, reality; the particular professional value orientations and ethical principles. The frame also defines and constitutes a collective identity or self, that is, who are professional members, and what do they represent. Typically they believe in and identify with the frame; they gain status and authority as well as material advantages through it. Members are expected to be loyal and committed – and typically are socialised and constrained to be loyal and committed – to the particular standpoint. Their general commitment to the profession or organisation means that members can be expected to provide testimony and support, often tacitly – and, as we see, through various rituals and discourses – to the expression of assumptions and judgements as well as actions of any given member. In sum, they are "like-minded" and like-committed (and this is a mutually shared assumption or belief), reinforcing the sense of commitment to the profession or professional organisation.

II. The standpoint or judgement frame is the basis on which members make judgements and take actions and, in general, know where they stand and, indeed, what stand to take (and what stand is expected of them). That is, within the frame, the actors can orient to commonly understood goods, determine what is good, or valuable (or bad), or what ought to be done (or avoided), or what one may properly endorse (or surely oppose). It is the basis of knowing right and wrong action, or the bases of admiration or respect of others in the profession, as well as the bases of contempt and shame (Taylor, 1989:27). In sum, the professional standpoint or judgement frame consists of a complex of values and norms, conceptions and beliefs on the basis of which problems are framed, defined, and analysed. Judgements can be made about how to solve problems, about what is right or wrong, and about how a member of the profession or professional organisation should conduct herself. In the case of medical professions, a part of the frame relates to ethical positions vis-à-vis patients as well as vis-à-vis colleagues. The professional frame thus defines particular standards of action to live up to – guidelines for acting in certain ways and expressing or realising certain values – in one's professional activities, for instance in interacting and dealing with patients, and, equally or more important, in their interactions and demonstrations of loyalties and commitments to one another and to the profession and professional organisation as a whole.

III. There are a variety of factors underlying members' commitment to the frame or standpoint, not least of which is "existential security". As Taylor (1989:27) suggests, if actors lose their commitment or identification, they would not know any more, for an important range of questions, what is good or worthwhile, or bad, or trivial and secondary; they would be "lost at sea". But the collective self or identity entails not only a standpoint, which is a basis for orientation, judgement and action, but an image and a status which matters to the members of the profession or professional organisation. It is a basis for them to command respect, even awe, and to exercise authority. In this sense it is a collective good or social capital (Bourdieu, 1991), a source of value not only for the collective as a whole but for its individual members.

IV. In acting and interacting, members of the profession or professional organisation may fail, or see others fail, in acting properly. Or outsiders may communicate and react critically from other moral standpoints (as next-of-kin do). Members may experience cognitive dissonance and distress, with respect to particular orientations, standards, expectations, and guidelines of their frame. However, the mere occurrence of dissonance conditions is not enough. As Billig (1982) points out, actors often experience dissonance-like situations, yet they do not experience distress or become engaged with the problematic cognitions. The most meaningful and stressful forms of dissonance arise in connection with cognitions or experiences which contradict the professional standpoint or frame (or particular judgements and actions derived from or closely associated with the frame). Such situations may become moments of crisis that not only challenge but give opportunity to the members of the collective to uphold the standpoint and principles that give them their identity, including their status and authority.

V. Specific cognitions – or the professional judgement frames from which they derive judgements, decisions, or actions in the hospitals – may be contradicted by information, communications, actions, and emotional states of some of the participants themselves (including next-of-kin or in some cases the patients themselves). Cognitive dissonance or imbalance dissonance occurs when an organisational belief, classification, judgement, or decision – that is derived from or generated within a particular professional and organisational order – is contradicted by subsequent information, another judgement, decision (there need not be a logical contradiction, but an interpretative or symbolic one). For instance: (1) The decision or belief that a patient is braindead is contradicted by data (observations, measurements, statements of others) that the patient appears alive rather than dead. (2) An established professional belief, judgement, or norm is contradicted by the way one acts. For example, a patient defined as dead is treated by medical personnel as if she is alive. (3) Nurses are engaged in situations where they deal with incompatible normative demands and conflicting emotions, and where their choices may lead to experiences of cognitive imbalance. They may be required to care for dead patients (braindead), who will be used for organ transplantation, and neglect living patients. (4) Nurses, who are expected to be caring and comforting, must often behave in detached ways in order to allocate their time and work efficiently. Whatever choice a nurse may make, for instance to devote time and attention to a particular task, may entail the neglect of other tasks, and the experience of dissonance as she is faced with negative consequences of her choice.

VI. Hospital professionals experience cognitive incongruence or dissonance in organisationally patterned ways. This relates also to the organisational division of labour and function – defining authority and responsibility – and to the occupational subcultures providing frames of meaning and assigning value to organisational experiences. In hospitals, for instance in intensive care units, attending physicians are required to make correct judgements and to act appropriately in relation to judgements of "life or death". Their responsibility and accountability – as result of their position or role in the organisation – is combined with situations where they lack complete information and control ("bounded control"). Data, experiences or messages that contradict professionally relevant cognitions and judgements can be highly problematic. Important values – and their own accountability with respect to what happens – are at stake. The problem in such action situations is one of assuring greater certainty, and stabilising cognitions.

VII. An argument developed in Chapter 8 is that the actors rely, adopt or develop organisational strategies to deal with dissonant or imbalance experiences. These are *collectively shared and institutionalised means for stabilising cognitions and resolving dissonance in organisational settings, such as hospitals.* This is under conditions where the sources of destabilisation cannot be simply corrected through direct action, either because such action is no longer feasible or is illegitimate (with risks of substantial sanctions for violations). Cognitive dissonance reduction or stabilisation is *biased*, tending to maintain in the face of challenge, critique, and threat the organisational and professional standpoint or frame with its particular conceptions and definitions of reality, beliefs and belief systems, its particular values and norms, and status and authority relationships. Members resolve dissonance in favour of their organisational and professional loyalties and commitments (to the collective standpoint) as opposed to the cognitive challenge or threat itself, whether this occurs in the form of actual performance failures, negative assessments or judgements (including those communicated by others).

VIII. Experience often fails to correspond to actors' plans or intentions, or to the institutional arrangements with which they organise and regulate their activities. Concrete action settings always entail flow and flux, irregularities, and disorder. This generates problems for cognitive stability and certainty. It is especially problematic in situations where actors in an organisation in their particular positions or roles are expected (and expect themselves) to make judgements and to act and to account for (and possibly defend) their actions (or the judgements on which they are based) in particular ways, according to the definitions and standards of a more or less well-defined professional judgement frame. Unintended consequences, irregularities, and disorder are often correlated with the introduction of new techniques and technologies, particularly radical ones.

As discussed in Chapters 6 and 8, new techniques and technologies tend to destabilise the professional standpoint by generating new problems and issues – which are disorienting or which create a sense of uncertainty and increased risk in the face of the problems and issues. The principles and guidelines of the professional frame may not indicate at least initially what is the proper conduct, what is right or wrong, or the fact that members have differing interpretations and arguments. Or questioning and critique comes from others outside the profession, challenging the judgement of the profession, or its leading members in the face of the new developments.

The Social Order of the Hospital

Social Order and Hospital and Professional Identities

A more or less shared judgement frame among the key professional groups, physicians and nurses, provides a systematic, inter-subjective basis for organising perceptions and guiding and regulating action and interaction in that order and for defining collective identity. The judgement or cognitive-normative frame (with its classification schemes, organising principles, and norms) is shared to a greater or lesser extent by key professional groups in the hospital as a basis for these actors to collectively construct and maintain (and also defend) a particular social order. This order is characterised by: (1) values oriented to helping clients achieve healthy states, or minimising illness and suffering; (2) a "science" (medical) knowledge frame along with specific technologies, and techniques, which are key components of the order; and (3) discourses and rituals that reinforce their beliefs in the medical framework and the hospital order. These core professions have a mission, or sacred duty, to serve the welfare of their patients (ideally never to exploit or cause harm to them), and to do this on the basis of possessing and applying "true" or scientific and clinical knowledge.

Anspach (1993:49) stresses the particular perspective and order of medical settings. The participants perceive their situation from more or less a specific vantage point: for instance, that physicians are responsible for making key medical determinations, and these are supposed to be carried out competently and in a trustworthy manner. There are life-and-death situations, death and suffering, dirty tasks. There is risk and danger of moral or ethical mistakes; illegalities can be committed; one can breach a key law or norm, or cross a boundary which brings dishonour, and exclusion, and disorder.

The order of the modern hospital, as in the case of other complex organisations, entails a number of more or less shared conceptions, symbols, classification schemes, and rules for defining situations, images of the organisation of themselves and of their clients, defining or specifying what are the significant concerns and dimensions involving the collective and its members (Burns and Flam, 1987):[159] (1) What type of situation is this? What is or should be going on here? (2) Who participates, who is included? Who shares in the identity of the organisation, and who is excluded? (3) What positions or roles do these participants have, what are their identities within the order? (4) What relationships do they have, for instance authority relations or superordinate/subordinate relations? What are the rights of control, obedience, differential access to resources? (5) What purposes, values, norms, etc. are supposed to orient actors, and are referred to in normative discourses, accounts, criticisms relating to what they do, what they should or should not do? (6) What activities, rituals, established discourses are considered right, proper, legitimate? (7) What are proper resources, tools, means, etc. (to some extent normatively regulated, to some extent "instrumental")? (8) What are the times, places, domains, or territories where they operate?

The shared frame in a modern hospital context includes collective representations and classificatory schemes applied in constituting and regulating patterns that make up the hospital order. The participating and knowledgeable professionals have a basis – in intersubjective ways – to define, interpret, and understand what they can and should do together, and the ways in which they are to do it, the reasons for doing it (or not doing it). They give accounts, make inquiries, and justify what they are doing or what is happening with reference to the common judgement frame. The frame also serves as a point of departure for legitimate critique and oppositions to particular actions, events, actors, or developments. *This shared frame of reference makes for solidarity in classifying (Douglas, 1987)*[160] *and in judging normatively.*[161] In other words, there is a not only a cognitive and normative intersubjectivity but solidarity, the everyday experience of solidarity in interactions. An individual participant feels in representational and moral harmony with other participants and feels more certain, secure, decisive, bolder in action, even in the face of outsiders or others who are truly "foreign" or who question the order. In a certain sense, cognitive imbalance and dissonance of the type that we have focused on here disturb, in some cases, threaten cognitive and normative solidarity – based on a shared judgement frame(s) for which the medical collective stands.

Such a frame provides key systems of classification. The importance of classifications in the regulation and maintenance of the hospital order can not be over-emphasised. Naming and defining biological matter as living, non-living, human or non-human, renewable or non-renewable, has organisational, ethical, and legal consequences in hospital settings (see Chapter 9). Classifications schemes thus are primary organisational devices in the maintenance of order.[162] A fundamental classification in any social order is the distinction between *the sacred and the profane* (Durkheim, 1912; Douglas, 1966). Through discourses and rituals, this basic distinction is maintained. This then allows for making other distinctions essential to the constitution and regulation of the social order.

A major system of classification in a hospital is that of categories of social actor, in particular the various health care personnel, their positions, statuses, and roles within the organisational set-up. There are also systems to classify patients,[163] diseases, states of aliveness or death. Labels stabilise social life in part through self-fulfilling processes, creating particular realities to which they apply, providing labels to which many people adjust or fit themselves, etc., not merely the medical personnel but patients and next-of-kin as well (Anspach, 1993; Douglas, 1987). In intensive care units, patients are in a highly transitional state, which optimally ends with the patient recovering from a critical condition. Patients "pass through" different statuses, for example living, comatose, and dead as well as intermediate liminal states. Physicians have the responsibility and authority to judge the passage of patients through these stages (also nurses participate). Thus, medical personnel, particularly physicians, have a strategic role as "social definers" of the status/position of patients, assuring that "proper" distinctions are being made, and proper actions are taken on the basis of these. Dissonance may arise in connection with these evaluations, judgements, and action. *Without this*

ordering on a cognitive level as well on the action level, there would be
the risk of an erosion of order and a confusing "sameness" with serious
professional, legal, and social consequences.

Many hospital situations entail critical matters of responsibility – as
in distinguishing a living from a dead person. The importance of
maintaining a cognitive and social order cannot be over-emphasised.[164]
Cognitive stabilisation has *anchoring or reference points* closely
associated with professional and organisational identities; these are at the
core of a cognitive complex including identity-giving roles and role
relationships, responsibilities and rights, and key norms and values,
matters we discuss below.

Key Referentials in Collective Identity

(1) The hospital is differentiated from other domains and institutional
arrangements by certain configurations of principles, rules, values, and
norms that give the hospital and its professionals their identities, their
core social relations, and their boundary(ies). These configurations do
more than give the order its particular identity; they are also a basis for
professional legitimacy and authority – and claims for support when it
comes to financing medical care and engaging in particular types of
research and treatment. These ingredients are central, even sacred, for
most professional members, and they cherish them deeply and are
prepared to defend them vigorously, to offer themselves for them
(Douglas, 1987).

(2) For both individual and collective actors, identity plays a major role
in organising and regulating their activities. An agent with a well-defined
identity knows how to act, how others are likely to respond, what can be
done in dealing with these responses. There is ontological security
(Wiley, 1994), that is, belief in one's standpoint, one's capacity to act
properly toward and to deal with others (Taylor, 1989). There is a secure
sense of self-confidence. Others orient and react to self in predictable
ways. And self in turn can make use of an established repertoire of
responses.[165] Moreover, being in a position to claim or refer to collective
identity – professional and/or organisational – is clearly advantageous
when it engenders high authority, status, prestige, public trust, and
legitimacy. Such cultural capital is the basis for a collective such as a
hospital and its core professionals to exercise power and influence vis-à-
vis others, in part defining situations and deciding agendas and discourses
as well as programs and plans of action. It is not suprising then that the
high status groups of a hospital enjoying authoritative and high-status

identities react strongly and emotionally when their core identities are challenged or threatened. For example, particular events, actions, developments, statements, or entire discourses suggest or witness the professional group or individual members as untrustworthy or even incompetent, contrary to their ideal images or identities. The collective, and its individual members, risk losing out in power, status, and legitimacy. If an identity is polluted or eroded – if physicians appear or are defined as "body snatchers" or as "businessmen", their patients, authorities, and the larger society are likely to change their orientations and behaviour vis-à-vis them, decreasing their influence or authority. Moreover, some of them may suffer a loss of belief in their own capabilities, a belief indispensable in acting self-confidently and self-righteously. In sum, there are practical reasons for maintaining or defending a high status identity and reacting strongly to challenges or threats to it. The stability of a judgement frame (along with its rules and schemes) is essential to "right behaviour" and depends on a variety of institutionalised cognitive, ritual, and discursive processes. That is, professionals in the organisation, in their positions and roles engage in cognitive and action/interaction processes that operate to maintain cognitive and interaction order.[166] They engage in various cognitive balancing and dissonance reducing processes to stabilise their self-images in the face of dissonant information or images: for instance, providing interpretations, redefinitions, presentation or re-presentation of actions and their outcomes, image-making, and impression management consistent with proper identity and self-definition. If a report, for example, reaches medical personnel that a trained physician or nurse has either intentionally or unintentionally (but incompetently) caused significant harm to a patient, they will tend to disbelieve the information, particularly if it comes from illegitimate or dubious sources, or is characterised by ambiguity. This and similar processes of cognitive stabilisation are examined in the following chapter.

Disturbances to Social Order and Challenges to Collective Identity

In any organisation there is always extraneous information, contradictory and ambiguous information, in a word "noise".[167] For instance: (1) there may be statements or communications that do not fit, or that challenge key beliefs and value orientations; (2) authority may be challenged; (3) actions may be taken by mistake; or out of ignorance, situational pressure, or adherence to contradictory goals. Any of these situations may result in contradictions with basic assumptions, conceptions, classifications, norms and values and the self-image of the organisation or its core professionals.[168] Insiders themselves sometimes behave in ways which contradict basic conceptions and principles of their social order. For instance, medical personnel may be compelled to perform acts – such as turning off life-sustaining equipment – that appear to harm or violate bodies or the health of patients. In this way, they might appear to dishonour the sanctity of life, or fail to live up to an image of dedication to the welfare of patients. They (or at least some of them) often recognise this themselves in that they activate rituals and discourses to correct or to stabilise cognitions consistent with the professional or hospital image.

Patients and next-of-kin can challenge and disrupt the order on a number of levels: they can question the substance of a decision; they may refuse to accept a diagnosis or prognosis; or particular actions taken. They may also direct critique and anger against the staff. They speak out and act in ways which disrupt or call into question the staff's self-conception and ethical position. They can challenge the social structure of doctor-patient relations or the professional prerogatives to dominate judgement and the decision-making process. Even without intending to do so, they introduce cognitive imbalance and dissonance into the situation, and must be dealt with, as part of the process of maintaining the social order of the hospital. For instance, the next-of-kin of a patient may complain that medical personnel are not doing their utmost and they are careless about the patient or they are not making use of available techniques. Or they may complain that the personnel, in particular the responsible physician(s), are incompetent or lack sufficient expertise. The hospital order would be disrupted unless measures are taken to buffer it from, or to deal with, such problems caused by "outsiders". [169]

The thoughts and actions of outsiders (next-of-kin as well as experts, mass media, politicians) are not fully predictably – and are certainly not under complete regulation and sanctioning from the hospital order.[170] Outsiders may raise questions or express beliefs, values, or emotions, or act in ways that contradict and disturb the hospital order – its collective representations, its authority relationships, its normative rules, among other things. Or they may call into question particular (scientific) judgements, or fundamental beliefs about the right ways to do things. In a variety of ways, they can cause dissonance and other cognitive disturbances with respect to key cognitions, expectations, beliefs, normative patterns, judgements or decisions. These are elements deriving from, symbolising, or representing the social order of the hospital: its particular medical frame or perspective, its normative principles and values, its authority and other institutional arrangements.

Disturbances to, and instability in, the cognitive and social order is not simply a personal problem for an individual member of the organisation. The problem is in many instances collective in that the shared judgement frame – or cognitive elements derived from or associated with it within the hospital order – are disturbed, challenged, threatened, and destabilised. Thus, fundamental challenges to medical authority or knowledge – on which the order depends heavily – are, therefore, major destabilising factors. Any criticism, inquiry, or anger directed against staff members for being indifferent or incompetent is likely to be disruptive. Why? Because it implies that they lack the proper professional value orientation and commitment. Either they are uninterested, unconcerned (therefore, not to be trusted) or they are incapable (and not to be trusted in another sense). For instance, when next-of-kin say that the staff is indifferent, cold, callous, they call into question the staff's self-image as healers and comforters. In such ways, outsiders can challenge professional self-image, their sense of competence, their sense of being ethical and trustworthy, and their operating rules regulating the expression of feelings and emotions about patients, "braindead", and "dead" (also see Anspach, 1993:162).

In sum, *the cognitive-normative solidarity of professionals in the hospital order is subject to disturbance and challenge, especially from outsiders, but even from persons within its own ranks.*[171] In the following chapter, we shall identify and analyse several of the strategies and processes whereby dissonance is resolved and cognitive stability maintained.

8 Resolving Dissonance Organisationally

Introduction

The previous chapter identified situations in hospitals where medical personnel (as well as next-of-kin) experience cognitive disturbance and imbalance, in particular in connection with dealing with braindead donors and organ retrieval. This chapter extends the research by articulating and applying the theoretical principle that *cognitive imbalance and dissonance in many key organisational situations are reduced or eliminated through organisational arrangements, and practices. This contributes to maintaining a stable, cognitive order and definition of the situation.* That is, professionals in hospitals, develop and utilise institutionalised means – discourses, rituals, and other practices – to assure routinely or in taken-for-granted ways information selectivity, re-interpretation, and re-framing the situation so as to stabilise key cognitions, beliefs, or judgements in the face of incongruous or dissonant information. Through such mechanisms, a cognitive component to which actors are committed – or the judgement frame in which it is part of a configuration or from which it derives – is stabilised even in the face of contradiction and disturbance.

The hospital situations on which the analysis focuses are those where there is no possibility of "correcting" cognitive imbalance through direct action, for instance by actually correcting "deviations" or "errors" or restructuring the environment (such imbalances could be eliminated in some objective sense). The judgements and decisions have taken place, action commitments have been made, and events have occurred. In a word, there is a *fait accompli*. Under such conditions, organisational arrangements, discourses, and rituals operate to resolve or minimise cognitive imbalance; these organisational components are identified in the first section. The following section discusses the centrality of cognitive balancing processes in relationship to social order. The final section discusses the possibility of extending the scope of the theory to explain cognitive imbalance and dissonance in other types of organisations, and the role of institutionalised means of resolving or minimising such imbalances. It is suggested that further research is needed on the role of institutionalised discourses, rituals, and organisational arrangements in maintaining cognitive stability in the face of destabilising events, developments, among others rapid technological change.

Organisational Means to Resolve or Reduce Cognitive Imbalance

Major cognitive balancing processes are well-known (Aronson, 1969; 1995; Festinger, 1957; Heider, 1958), particularly *information selectivity, re-interpretation, and re-definition or re-framing*. In our formulation, these are embedded in organisational arrangements and processes, which operate to reduce cognitive imbalance and, in particular, dissonance (in some cases to preclude or prevent such experiences arising) and to stabilise key cognitions and cognitive frames.

(a) *Information selectivity.* Organisational information systems, procedures, and discourses reduce or eliminate cognitive imbalance, that is stabilise cognitions or judgements, by selecting (and also excluding) information. In general, information selection and structuring is one of the most common organisational mechanisms for stabilisation. Certain information is given legitimacy and other data, for instance that contributing to cognitive imbalance, is defined as illegitimate or inappropriate. Or members regularly activate or consider additional information in order to countervail or minimise imbalance experiences.

(b) *Re-interpretation.* Routine organisational statements and discourses provide consonant interpretations of otherwise incongruous or dissonant information. Data that is contradictory is re-conceptualised, re-interpreted, or re-perceived to be consistent with the main judgement or belief (or in some cases is defined as not applying). Thus, *"meaning" is structured, or even transformed,* for example in a statement such as the following: "We are certain the patient is dead, that is braindead, after our determinations. Brain death is a scientific concept and procedures for determining brain death are reliable. Although the patient exhibits some 'indications of life', they are misleading".

(c) *Re-definition of the situation; definition of non-relevancy.* Again, established organisational discourses define certain situations, experiences, types of data as not relevant, thereby reducing or eliminating imbalance experiences. The importance or relevance of the dissonant situation is reduced. For example, the nurse who stresses that, "This is not my (or our) responsibility. I'm not the one who made the judgement; it was my superior, therefore I am not accountable". (This is, of course, *a highly legitimate means* within many organisations to reduce or resolve cognitive imbalance.) Or one can distance oneself from emotional engagement through professional language, use of technologies, particular techniques or procedures. Normative discourses – and account giving – are widely used for cognitive balancing within organisational contexts. This is a public or collective way of redefining the salience or connectivity

– or their opposites – of the self, whether individual or collective, to the situation.

In the following section, I will focus specifically on organisational discourses, design, and rituals that minimise or resolve cognitive imbalance through information selectivity, re-interpretation, and re-definition or re-framing.

Dissonant Reducing Discourses: Socially Defining (or Re-defining) the Situation

Discourse is a complex communicative act, a structure of spoken or written language as in conversations, interviews, speeches, and texts of various types and forms.[172] Meaning is not conveyed by a single sentence or utterance but through more complex formulations and exchanges on the basis of which the participants define the context and express beliefs and expectations and commitments. They demonstrate their common knowledge. Discourses are a key factor in the continuous production and reproduction of meanings. Of course, as the analyses suggests, discourses as all communications are a part of a larger framework of interaction and social structure (Burns and Dietz, 1997; Burns and Flam, 1987, Collins, 1988:321).

Through discourses, actors create an operative definition of the situation and thus have a basis for acting together – in part through a commonly held social rule and role knowledge entailing rules and paradigmatic examples and situational knowledge of how to enact various social rules and roles (Brulle, 1994:101; Burns and Flam, 1987). *Through discursive and cognitive closure, social order can be established and maintained, a particular reality defined and stabilised.* In Foucault's terms, such closure defines "regimes of truth" on the basis of which actors orient to one another, make judgements, and interact. Foucault (1972:131), arguing on a more macroscopic level than OTC, argues:

> Each society has its regime of truth, its "general politics" of truth: that is, the types of discourse which it accepts and makes function as true; the mechanisms and instances which enable one to distinguish true and false statements, the means by which each is sanctioned; the techniques and procedures accorded value in the acquisition of truth; the status of those who are charged with saying what counts as true.

Applying such a notion to organisations, Brulle (1994:100-101) points out:

> Symbolic closure has two effects. The first effect is the creation of discourse, forms of knowledge, and comprehensible social reality, which enables the production of social organisation. In addition, while

affirming one reality, symbolic closure must inherently reject the other alternative definitions of the situation. Thus the second effect of closure is the exclusion of the alternative realities, and the creation of subjugated discourses.

Discourses as institutionalised communications, written or oral, are defined and understood within a particular organisation, collectivity, or field of social action (Bourdieu, 1991; Brulle, 1995; Burns and Sutton, 1995; Ellingson, 1995). Discourses represent or articulate judgements: reality judgements, value judgements, action judgements or decisions. For instance, they concern the definition and nature of social reality: what are problems or types of problems. They also provide explanations, and may contain arguments in the form of claims, images, or tropes combined in a more or less coherent manner and intended to persuade others through an appeal to logic, fact, belief, emotion, or external authority (Ellingson, 1995). Finally they convey what are the right and proper solutions, what is to be done or not done (Sutton, 1998).

There are established rules (often implicit) for articulating any given discourse, its form, its content; for determining which actors may articulate the discourse (and who may not), who may be privy to it, and so forth. In the medical literature, there are a number of studies of particular discursive activities in hospital settings (see especially Anspach, 1993; Fox, 1988, 1989; Machado, 1997; Waitzkin, 1989; Waitzkin et al., 1994) that address ambiguity, dissonance, contradiction and conflicts. They accomplish this by conveying meaning, providing definitions or redefinitions of the situation. They also interpret and explain events – for instance, they explain away or minimise the importance of unpleasant or dissonant-producing facts. This relates to the basic notion that discourses are conveyers of meaning. A few major types of cognitive balancing discourse can be identified in hospital settings and are outlined below. These are types that I identify as playing a substantial role in cognitive as well as social stabilisation.

(1) *Discourses   that frame and stabilise cognitions in connection with brain death*: The problems of cognitive imbalance in a "charged" social context are not merely cognitive in character but typically normative and emotional, for instance the question of finding the normatively or morally correct action and the proper management of emotions. The traces of people's memories, orientations, habits, etc. toward, for example, a person who had been alive creates problems of *re-orientation and change of relationships and roles, when that person dies.* Concerning death settings in hospitals, Glaser and Strauss (1965:113-114) point out:

When a patient has just died, people who see the corpse rather soon thereafter tend, under certain conditions, to behave almost as if the patient were alive and aware of its imminent death. Temporarily the deceased is regarded virtually as a sentient person... Relatives, immediately after the patient's death, often speak or caress him as if he were alive. Although they know he is dead, they act as if he knew what they were saying and doing, because his death is so recent. Staff members rarely speak to or caress the corpse, but in a lower key they sometimes act as much like kinsmen. The tendency to treat a recently deceased kinsman as if he (*she*) were still alive is reinforced by the nurses' or physicians' efforts to protect family members, arranging appearances so that the deceased person resembles his former self.

Health care personnel in intensive care units articulate special discourses to "re-arrange" cognitively dissonant situations, such as that the maintenance of the braindead entails. One distinct discursive form that has emerged is the development of *the two-phase concept and discourse of death* (see Chapter 6 and also Younger, 1992:571):

An even greater problem with the term "brain death", arises, from the lingering doubt that individuals with brain death are really dead. Hence, even physicians are sometimes heard to say that the patient "suffered brain death" one day and "died" the following day (Veatch:1993:18).

Health professionals regularly use the term "braindead" to describe patients that are legally dead, and refer to them as "dead" only when the ventilator is turned off after the organs have been removed. Arnold and Youngner (1993:267) report:

...the observation that many health professionals (and most journalists) describe "braindead" patients as having "died" only after either life-support devices or organs are removed, suggests that many persons disagree with, or are, at minimum, ambivalent about the conceptual status of the persons whose brains have ceased functioning but whose hearts continue to beat.

The time of the death noted on death certificates is when the heart stopped, not when the patient is diagnosed as braindead. The latter time is regularly the one noted on death certificates (Youngner et al., 1989; Youngner, 1992:2160). As a leading researcher in this area puts it:

In my experience, the time of the death noted on death certificates is when the heart stopped, not when the patient was diagnosed as braindead. This situation is not desirable. If we want to convince the general public that organ donors are indeed dead, we should call them that. The solution? Not surprisingly, I have heard many people suggest that we should simply stop using the term braindead...Terms like "harvest" and "braindead" persist because they reflect uncomfortable feelings and conceptual ambiguities inherent in transplantation...The use of those loaded words stubbornly persist because they express ambiguities and grisly associations that are psychologically valid. To order them away would be an act of futility, or worse, could be counterproductive. The use of these terms, like jokes (and there are many jokes about transplantation), facilitates *a socially acceptable release of fears and ambivalence about transplantation that allows rather than undermines our acceptance of some of its more horrifying aspects* (Youngner, 1992:2160).

If one asks medical personnel in this setting about the moment of death, they will explain rationally that it is "brain death". But their actual discourses and practices indicate another cognitive and practical reality.

(2) *Authoritative discourses*: Numerous discourses in hospital settings refer to the authority of physicians, medical knowledge and technology, "solid, reliable information" from particular instruments (providing "data" and "answers"), or "medical expertise" in supporting a particular judgement, decision, intervention, etc. The key to making discourses authoritative is that they are made by persons socially defined or certified as authoritative; also, that there are no bona fide alternatives (medical personnel typically maintain a common front; disagreements among them are particularly disruptive to medical authority and order).

The scientific judgement frame – and the discourses articulating it – are a major basis for establishing and maintaining cognitive stability within medical settings. In general, scientific-medical discourses among hospital personnel are used to define and legitimise statements, actions, rituals that resolve imbalance or dissonant experiences concerning death, organ extraction, etc. Such constitutive or meta-discourses are supported by the authority of particular physicians, the medical profession, and the array of medical schools, hospitals, *Nobel prizes, and other signs of social recognition and status, etc.*

Examples of particular constitutive discourses that define and legitimise tools to resolve actual or potential cognitive imbalance are the Harvard and Pittsburgh Protocols as well as particular laws and regulations, circulars, etc.[173] These protocols legitimise judgements and particular procedures, serving thereby to minimise cognitive imbalance among medical personnel. They are also referred to by medical personnel in their discourses on brain death and organ transplantation. In short, they consist of routine, everyday professional discourses for dealing with and resolving specific instances of cognitive imbalance and dissonance in clinical settings.

In general, medical discourses are used to define the situation, such as the "patient is dead, because..." (referring to tests or indications). As Zussman (1992: 149) points out, "Dead is when doctors say she's dead". A definitional discourse may redefine organ extraction or harvesting as saving someone else's life with this extraction of organs.

The authority of physicians – and of hospital personnel in general – vis-à-vis patients (and their friends and next-of-kin) is based on discourses and actions socially defining the situations. Physicians are defined as authoritative, knowledgeable, trustworthy. As long as physicians and other hospital personnel as well as others can convince patients and next-of-kin of their expert knowledge, their trustworthiness, the rightness and propriety of their authority, the likelihood of deference to them – and compliance with their strictures and demands – is maintained. This shared definition of reality enables them – with support or acquiescence from others (other patients, the public, police, etc.) – to maintain the hospital order and to deal with problems of disruptive deviance.

(3) *Dismissal and de-legitimising discourses*: A common type of discourse are those that disqualify lay persons including next-of-kin who question or refuse to accept a diagnosis, prognosis, or medical report, as "uninformed", or as "emotional", "unrealistic", irrational", etc. Typically, dismissive discourses counter and balance statements and stories that question or challenge the authority of physicians and the medical technologies and techniques which are defined as the basis of most medical determinations.

Next-of-kin of a dying or dead person often have difficulty interpreting – at least with any security – their own observations and the information they receive from medical personnel. (Of course, there is considerable information that they do not gain access to or are incapable of interpreting.) They turn naturally to medical authority for clarification, for answers to their questions motivated by dissonant experiences and uncertainty. Such authorities in turn provide an explanation or interpretation of these experiences – for instance, that there is no inconsistency between the definition of the person as dead and the perception of the patient as apparently alive. Or they utilise normalised statements to reassure next-of-kin that their braindead relative is, indeed, dead, that she is not suffering, that she does not feel anything when organs are removed – and that the removal of organs will result in good for others. There are numerous more or less institutionalised formulations to address discordant information, to deny or exclude information, or to re-interpret it, or redefine situations so that dissonant experiences may be ignored or considered irrelevant.

Major processes of definition and interpretation in most life and death situations in hospitals are directed or managed in large part by physicians. Nurses rely on this social fact in communicating, for example, with next-of-kin. They refer to the doctor's opinion or judgement. Next-of-kin themselves turn to medical authority, often first a nurse, but ultimately a doctor, to be informed (physicians serving as ultimate authorities, "judges of last resort"). Even many non-physicians (nurses, patients, and next-of-kin) largely accept the medical science ethos, its machines and tests as key factors in defining problems as well as solutions and in dispelling uncertainties and anxieties, for instance in addressing the question why a person declared dead still appears to be alive. As one of our interviewees (nursing assistant, Sweden) put it:

> I'm not sure what happened, but the braindead patient, who was perhaps not absolutely braindead, but practically so, began dying (in terms of heart and respiratory functions), and the alarm of the ventilator was activated and started to sound. I said to the relatives that the device was not functioning properly.

Note that the statement to the relatives provides a re-interpretation of what was happening, referring to a technology of which the relatives are ignorant. It also illustrates the emergence of new types of discourse in connection with brain death, namely *reinterpreting the significance of physical manifestations*, that prior to the concept of brain death were regarded as signs of life. These serve to constitute and stabilise the cognition – and collective representation – that braindead persons are in fact dead. [174]

(4) *Labelling and jokes*: The use of derogatory names and stories, jokes, complaints, etc. in medical settings is widely reported (Fox, 1988; 1989). For instance, there is a well-developed gallows humour and hyper-realistic "horror stories" about what can and does go wrong in the treatment of patients (Fox, 1989: 155). Fox (1988:579-580) reports, "Counterphobic and ironic, infused with bravado and self-mockery, often impious, defiant, and macabre, it [the humour] closely resembles what Freud termed 'gallows-humour', and the front-lines-of-the-battlefield humour ...It occurs most frequently and floridly in situations where medical professionals are under an unusual or extreme amount of stress, and it most characteristically centres on medical uncertainty, the limitations of medical knowledge, medical errors, and the side effects of medical and surgical interventions, the failure to cure, sex and sexuality, and, above all, death. It is epitomised, for example, in the names that oncologists have given to some of the chemotherapy protocols that they use to treat cancer; SCARY, CRAB, CURE, POMP." Such humour, we suggest (also, see Fox (1988: 580), is an in-group, emotional code through which medical professionals confront, express, release, and handle some of the deepest, most powerful and threatening feelings of cognitive dissonance or

imbalance, anxiety, and distress connected with their work. Fox (1988: 580-581) reports:

> Nurses and physicians speak and write of the "dread graft-versus-host disease reaction" to bone marrow transplantation, for example, or of "rescuing" patients after they have undergone sublethal doses of total body irradiation', and of "harvesting" organs for human transplantation. Coded into such phrases is their collective chagrin about the macabre nature of some of the activities in which they professionally engage, and about the amount of risk, suffering, and even harm to which they subject patients through their supposedly therapeutic interventions. The fact that such terms not only are used in face-to-face medical and nursing discussions, but also are standard vocabulary in professional publications, printed as if they were neutrally scientific terms, suggests that their relationships to medical stress is not as explicitly recognised by doctors and nurses.

Fox (1988:580-581) also refers to the use of initials as well as euphemisms:

> The term "end-stage renal disease", usually abbreviated ESRD in the journals is an example. Calling it "end-stage" rather than "terminal" kidney disease is perhaps more accurate in an era when hemodialysis and/or renal transplantation can keep a patient whose kidneys no longer function indefinitely alive; and referring to it as ESRD saves spoken time and printed space. But, in addition, it protects physicians and nurses from being constantly, verbally reminded that patients in this state are incurably ill, and that, at the present time, all that medicine can do for them is to "rescue" them continually from otherwise death and "maintain" them (as the medical expression goes) by means of so-called "half-way technology".

Jokes, complaints, expressions of "righteous anger" are also directed against those who disrupt professional work, in particular by challenging the profession's authority, status, sacred symbols (Collins, 1988: Chapter 6).[175] These express and also reinforce a shared judgement frame, with its collective representation of a right and proper social reality, a moral and symbolic world, and also intensify common feelings among themselves (at the expense of others), they enhance their solidarity and common identity. The symbolic reality created is the social identity of those taking part – their distinctiveness from others, their special authority and status in relation to patients, next-of-kin, the public, mass media, etc.

(5) *Success discourses.* Physicians may engage in a type of "scientific magic" which appear to reflect or express medical scientific ways of thinking and acting, yet serve to define medical innovations as successful – *even in the face of dissonant information or knowledge.* Fox (1989:195-

197) reports on the formulation of success stories in connection with the process and reporting of medical research and the development of innovations in medicines and techniques. This is manifested in a powerful predisposition to focus exuberantly on the positive features of a promising new drug or a new technique and to ignore or downplay their limitations and potentially harmful side effects, especially during the early stages of its experiment-to-therapy trajectory, and only later in the therapeutic innovation cycle – with some reflection and greater sobriety – to openly acknowledge limitations and potentially harmful side effects (Fox, 1989:196). Fox (1989:196) points out:

> There is no inherent biological reason why the discovery of the beneficial actions of a new drug should precede the identification of its disadvantages and contra-indications. Nor are there objective scientific grounds for investigators to be "surprised" and "disappointed" – as they often state that they are in the medical literature – when they encounter what they term the "vexing problem" of the undesirable secondary effects of an otherwise "remarkably effective" drug. Quite the contrary, no all-therapeutic, side-effect-free therapy of any sort has ever been found, and there are solid scientific grounds for assuming that none ever will be.

Through such mechanisms, physician/researchers maintain a horizon of hope even in the face of contrary information and keep the therapeutic innovation cycle in perpetual motion; they persevere in the face of a variety of dissonant messages and results, setbacks, and uncertainty that clinical investigation entails.

This pattern of development is an integral to the belief in medical progress – and physicians' central role in this – and motivates them to look for and try improved ways of preventing, treating, and managing disease. There is a persistent belief – and commitments and actions based on the belief – in the possibility of discovering a beneficent "wonder drug" or true "magic bullet". Dissonant reducing discourses contribute to maintaining the belief in the face of limitations and drawbacks that might create doubts and dissatisfaction about the initially high expectations. In this way, the impetus to continue the search – and a true believer mentality in trying to mobilise financial and other resources – for another new, "better" drug, repeating the therapeutic innovation cycle is maintained. And so on, again and again (Fox, 1989:196-197).

Thus, when a procedure – operation, treatment, research approach, etc. – fails or does not turn out as expected, this does not necessarily lead to a questioning or impugning the validity of the procedure, or the perspective in back of it. Rather, the problem or issue is re-framed through particular discourses. Belief in the procedure or approach remains "true". It was simply not carried out correctly, or was not carried far enough; or "forces" interfered with and counteracted it (Collins, 1988: 280).

Organisational Arrangements, Positions, and Props to Minimise or Reduce Cognitive Imbalance and Dissonance

(1) *Organisational structure and "spacing".* One of the main organisational measures in reducing or preventing cognitive imbalance is to separate potentially clashing (incongruous or dissonant) domains or procedures into discrete parts. "Spacing" manoeuvres, both in time and space, are classical organisational devices to structure and articulate different and even incongruous rule systems in organisational aggregates. In general, a typical organising principle or measure entails separating one domain of activity (domain 1) from another (domain 2), if the rules and procedures relating to conditions and activities in these domains are incongruous or incompatible. Thus, (1) may be the domain of the living, and (2) that of the dead. And social roles – moral conceptions and values as well as discourses – differ substantially. In domain 1 the physicians are "keepers", while in (2) they are the "reapers", the "organ harvesters".

Thus, cognitive imbalance is reduced by creating distinct, separate domains or settings and roles. Often it is claimed that the division of labour is motivated by instrumental rationality, for instance increasing effectiveness or efficiency, etc. But, according to the perspective we are offering here, *this division operates to reduce cognitive imbalance in situations where clarity, boundary maintenance, etc. are of critical importance* – where actors in some organisational positions are responsible for decisions, judgements, and actions taken.[176]

In general, organisational designers establish a set-up, for instance particular institutional arrangements as well as architecture so as to minimise the possibilities of cognitive imbalance, and thereby contribute to stabilising *a particular judgement frame.* This is accomplished partly through the familiar devices of emphasising clear goals, clear boundaries, explicit distribution of time, space and authority, and bounded jurisdiction of function (who does what, how, when, where, and for what purposes (Burns and Flam, 1987)). But, in part, through ritual, discourses, and utilisation of a number of props (as discussed below). In one neurosurgical unit where one of us has made observations and conducted interviews, the braindead donor (before the organ extraction) was separated from the deeply sedated or in coma patients, etc., that is the "living" (see Machado (1990) concerning the principle of organising in ways to reduce risk and cognitive imbalance or dissonance in risky situation).

One systematic arrangement for coping with potential cognitive and emotional disturbances is through the use of professional objectifying practices which focus as much as possible on body parts and organs and on the technical procedures for dealing with them (for instance, in the face of the dramatic circumstances of brain death and organ removal, medical personnel avoid practices and discourses in relation to braindead patients that appear alive and human in many respects). In her report on Swedish conditions, Sanner (1991:162) cites a nurse:

> One can behave very respectful towards the patient before. When they open [the donor] it comes a phase that for the relatives must be terribly disrespectful. It looks like a slaughter board. It is not respectful, but it can still be so for those standing there. They do not experience the same thing as an outsider. Later you seal the skin and suddenly it is a person there again. What is really respect? It is, to be technical, and this is valid for all operations and often what saves the life of a patient. *It is, not seeing the patient in what one does (I do) because perhaps then one could become stirred by feelings. It is important to keep distance.*

In general, medical personnel utilise a number of standard methods and procedures to protect themselves from painful realities and feelings. In this way, the participating medical personnel avoid becoming emotionally involved. As one Swedish nurse stated, "I no longer think of them [potential cadaver organ donors] as people but as objects for salvaging parts".[177]

The clinical language and perspective, even more so the medical scientific one, reinforces objectification and the authority of those who have the knowledge and competence not only to use this language but to make judgements and decisions on the basis of a clinical/scientific frame. The representation of the case, in particular in the journal, follows routine rules that realise objectification of patients: short description, chief complaint, history of illness, medical plan etc. Moreover, there are typically rules, procedures, and discourses to regulate and explain the critical boundary and passages between the domains of life and death. For instance, in the case of life and death situations, this is to assure that one is not causing – or has not caused through incompetence or moral inadequacy – the transition or passage from living to death.

(2) *Formal specialist roles to deal with dissonant situations.* One example of the use of specialisation to deal with problems of cognitive imbalance (and acquiring necessary expertise in managing these problems) is the creation of specialists who deal with organ procurement or extraction. They learn a particular perspective and particular discourses to deal with heart-beating cadavers. In this way, many of the problems that medical

personnel experience in the face of braindead "patients' are systematically (not only technically but social psychologically) handled.

In the "Medical News" of the Journal of the American Medical Association (1985:3287) this was brought up:

> The institution of systematic procurement programs has done more than set up systems within a hospital; it has also removed some of the emotional burden from hospital staff members. Those in the procurement team are taught to recognise that beating heart donors are, in fact, legally dead, and that organ retrieval is a positive rather than a harmful act.

Another instrument of an organisational character has been the creation of the special role of the transplantation nurse or transplantation co-ordinator, who contributes to defining ambiguous situations and to resolving dissonance. As one nurse (interviewee, Sweden) expressed it:

> Before the time of the co-ordinators, when a possible donor appeared it was very confusing, I did not know where to call, what to do. After that the rules became clear and it is very easy.

Many organisational measures entail, then, the creation of specialised groups (e.g. organ extractors), mediating positions (e.g. transplantation co-ordinator), emotional outlets (personnel meetings to ventilate problems), and socially centred in organisational rituals, redefinitions of the situation, and discourses that operate to resolve or minimise cognitive imbalance.

(3) *Organisational and professional practices and props.* A variety of organisational and professional props are utilised to clearly define (and distinguish) key medical situations and encounters, and thereby contribute to stabilisation of judgement frames. Medical examination rooms are characterised by a number of props which clearly define the situation and the appropriate orientations and feelings and exclude other orientations and feelings from occurring (or below the surface of consciousness): for instance, the generally white or green room; the stainless steel and leatherette examining table fitted out with white or green crepe chapter sheeting; its medical cabinet, through whose glass door instruments, bandages, and medications are visible; its sink, over which hang special soap and paper towel dispensers; and its occasional set of medical instructions, etc. defines to the physician, nurse, and patient that the setting is a scientific, medical one, where, however intimate a physician or nurse with a patient may be, professionally relevant and competent examinations are the only concern and are to be carried out with appropriate decorum (Fox, 1988:579). Another contextualising prop used

in the operating room is the routine procedure of draping the patient on the table – covering all parts of the patient's body except the specific area on which the surgeon works (Fox, 1988:579).[178]

Organisational procedures (including technical rituals using medical tests and equipment) serve to collectively define (and to assure) that proper consideration and respect are shown patients, even those who have died, or that a patient judged as dead is, indeed, dead.[179] Our interviews (but also reports in the literature (Sanner, 1991, among others), particularly in the case of nurses) indicate deep concerns about turning off life-support devices. Intensive care units develop various routines relating to the utilisation of devices that operate to prevent or minimise experiences of cognitive imbalance. For example, one of our interviewees in Sweden indicated that at her unit they regularly shut off the electrocardiograph (ECG) (that would indicate heart function and beat) before they take away "life" support equipment that maintains the "braindead" person. In this way, the personnel avoid the cognition or experience that they are doing something harmful to a living person, which would be incompatible with their clinical orientation and self-image.

The distinctions between discourse, ritual, organisational props and arrangements are analytical. Typically, they are combined in ongoing processes of producing and maintaining definitions of reality, particular meanings and meaning complexes. Thus, in medical encounters between physicians and patients, props as well as rituals and standardised discourses are apparent.

Re-Structuring Experience Through Organisational Rituals

Ritual is a type of patterned or *institutionalised symbolic action*, collectively defined and constituted within a group or organisation.[180] It consists of words, gestures, and actions and use of objects and artefacts to express a conception, symbolic meaning, feeling or sentiment within a group or collectivity ((Bell, 1992; Bosk, 1980; Burns and Laughlin, 1979; Chapman, 1983; Collins, 1988; Fox, 1989; Turner, 1991; Wolf, 1988).[181] Ritual entails two or more persons meeting or coming together, engaging in particular actions, or procedures according to a particular social grammar or complex of rules. Ritual focuses collective attention and mood and activates or generates a shared symbolic reality (Collins, 1988: Chapter 6), in our case here a hospital or particular clinical settings. When ritual is being performed, members of the group recognise the action, understand its meaning or the message that it expresses or its meaning.

While ritual may be employed in a variety of situations and

problems, we are interested here in rituals that minimise tensions and distress from cognitive contradiction or imbalance – *and do this in non-discursive (and non-rationalised) ways.*[182] This explains in part its persistence in highly "rationalised" settings such as hospitals. Hospital rituals are embedded to a significant degree in the schedules, procedures, and practices of a hospital (Bosk, 1980:177; Fox, 1989:155). For instance, there are "occupational rituals" inherent in such meetings as attending to patients, medical rounds, consultation, case conferences, and mortality and morbidity conferences, at which physicians discuss and analyse patient cases, the problems of making a proper diagnosis, and prescribing treatment for their patients (Fox, 1989:155). Fox (1989:155-156) points out: "These meetings involve more than intellectual, scientific, and technical exchanges about patient management. Built into them, Bosk (1980) shows, are ceremonial patterns of behaviour that "allow physicians to dramatise, to teach, and to remind themselves and their colleagues of their sense of what it means to be a physician", and that "assist them in managing uncertainty, making treatment decisions, and evaluating outcomes". Similarly, ritual aspects are observable in nurses' admission and discharge of patients, change of shift reporting, medical aseptic practices, and post-mortem care (Fox, 1989:156; Wolf, 1988). Indeed, nurses in their training are typically instructed to perform their task-lists as if performing a ritual, minimising the number and variety of decisions that must be made and communicating through actions vis-à-vis others, particularly outsiders, that one is devoted and efficient (Menzies, 1970).

Medical personnel structure many of their experiences through organisational rituals and routines (utilising in many instances medical technologies). For instance, the medical encounter between physician and patient is organised in several more or less standard formats (Waitzkin, 1989:228) entailing ritual activity. Rituals become one of the most important devices to "re-structure" experience or alter the experience of situations or events[183] (Bell, 1992; Burns and Laughlin, 1979; Collins, 1988; Handelman, 1995; Turner, 1969). Through institutionalised rituals within hospitals, professionals structure their own experiences and the experiences of their clients and avoid or negate particular dissonant or dis-equilibrating information by producing or constructing new or different experiences.

Physicians (along with other high status professions) are particularly effective at establishing and maintaining the *ritual impressiveness* of the stage on which they encounter their clients and others (Collins, 1988: 205). Collins (1988:205-206) points out:

They utilise their high rank and considerable power and authority to exercise great control over the stage settings in which they meet their clients and others.... Doctors meet their patients in carefully prepared consulting rooms, make their entrance through their own private back corridors, and tightly manage the information which gives them control of defining the reality of the situation.

One part of the structuring of ritual conditions of self-presentation is to arrange to have assistants or nurses to take care of the "dirty work". In this way, they also avoid potential contamination or degradation. In general, physicians are in an advantageous position to initiate and take part in rituals on their own terms, with the greatest physical resources for appearing impressive and avoiding degrading or debilitating activities.

In the particular medical settings that we have investigated, rituals are apparent in showing deep concern about patients, confronting the dead, expressing authority, practising self-criticism without undermining authority, or showing deference.[184] Among major identifiable rituals of interest are the following: (1) *Rituals of caring*. There are variety of rituals performed by nurses such as fixing pillows, touching the patient, taking temperature, writing down information. These rituals communicate concern and caring – thus conveying the identity and normative orientation of nurses. This may be done in the face of pressures that prevent nurses from doing very much for any patient. They must allocate their scarce time and attention. In short, they must be effective and also detached to a considerable degree. The rituals redefine, for example, instances or experiences (those of the nurses as well as next-of-kin and conscious patients) of lack of medical attention and concern as ones of concern and commitment to the patients. (2) *Rituals of authority and deference*. There are various rituals to demonstrate and to reinforce respect to doctors (Anspach, 1993; Chapman, 1983:19) as well as to nurses with authority.[185] These are important in maintaining the order of norms and authority in the face of challenge or potential challenge, for instance next-of-kin questioning the judgement of a physician concerning the status of a dying patient. (3) *Rituals of self-criticism and abasement*. At mortality and morbidity conferences, senior (attending) surgeons publicly and ceremonially "abase themselves" before their peers and subordinates (Bosk, 1980; Fox, 1989:155). They point out their own mistakes, that they have made mistakes in the handling of patient's cases under discussion, typically explaining why it might have been better to take some other course of action and noting the lessons that have been learned (Fox, 1989:155).[186] (4) *Rites de passage*. There are a variety of such rituals in dealing with the dead or dying in medical settings (Fox, 1989; Chapman, 1983, among others).

Of particular interest to us have been socially established procedures to cope with cognitive dissonance and distress in dealing with the braindead organ donors, or the patients who are to be allowed to die. It is not an uncommon procedure to wait for a patient's heart to stop after the ventilator support is removed (that is, waiting for a type of "second death"). As one of our interviewees (nurse, Sweden) put it, "No organ extraction was to be performed. We disconnected the ventilator and waited beside the bed of patient until the heart stopped beating", as if the moment of the cardiac arrest would be a more genuine or true moment of the death. It is then that traditionally the individual makes the transition from life to death. Customarily, the next-of-kin is expected to be present to give the last farewell to the dying person, and the whole moment has a atmosphere of deference and respect. Not being present at the "moment of death" can be distressing for the relatives since for many this moment has assumed a sacred and fundamental quality. Its absence is disturbing.

One of the institutionalised means for reducing cognitive imbalance in connection with death is through rituals of passage that socially or collectively define the patient as at rest. One common pattern in hospitals are post-mortem rituals or rituals of closure, clearly defining that the end has come such as "dressing the body" of the deceased in a proper way (Fox, 1988, 1989; Wolf, 1991). One of our interviewees reports that in the case of braindead non-donors in the ICU, the devices are shut off, the "patient" is cleaned and prepared. Flowers may be placed on the body by a nurse, and next-of-kin admitted. After a patient has died (and organs possibly removed), there is nothing more to do medically. Through the rituals, the personnel show respect, care and consideration. A number of studies have pointed out the importance of post-mortem rituals, for example:

> All members of the team withdrawing support felt a need to acknowledge or to commemorate the passing of life by more than the pronouncement of death by the supervising CCM physician. The ICU nurses reported that when a patient dies in the ICU, the bedside nurse often participates directly in the post-mortem care. It may be that this physical task allows the care giver an opportunity to accept death and come to psychological closure. Some suggested the observance of an analogous ritual in the OR, such as a brief prayer, eulogy by clergy or a "moment of silence" for all present (De Vita et al., 1993a: 376).

> Operating room personnel - nurses, were uncomfortable with the removal of life support in the OR, where usually every measure is taken to prevent death... They felt that strict supervision was necessary to prevent inappropriate removal of support and to ensure that support be removed humanely and without performing active euthanasia (De Vita et al., 1993b:135).

The ICU nurses and CCM physicians felt a strong need to remain with the cadaver out of respect for the deceased and shared a sense that leaving would constitute abandonment of the patient (De Vita et al., 1993a:377).

An essential characteristic of ritual (and ritualised behaviour) – that to a high degree accounts for its effectivity and cultural persistence – is that it enables actors to collectively handle dissonant and stressful situations in a non-discursive (i.e. non-verbalisable) way. A variety of hospital rituals – whether they occur among physicians, nurses, or other personnel in the ward or clinical unit, operating room, laboratory, or conference room – appear to cope with some of the problems of cognitive imbalance, dissonance, ambiguity and uncertainty and the tensions and distress that these can elicit. The contradictions and cognitive disturbances are not of any sort whatever but those relating to essential features of what a hospital – and its core professionals – do, represent, and stand responsible for. They provide physicians, nurses, and patients with collective ways of organising perceptions and feelings as well as institutionalised strategies to reduce or eliminate cognitive imbalance – or potential imbalance – arising in connection with dealing with the sick, dying, and dead and with challenges or threats to authority and status relationships in the hospital context.

Organisation Mechanisms, Cognitive Stabilisation, and Social Order

OTC stresses the cognitive dimension of organisational processes, in particular the fundamental role that cognition, and micro-processes generally, play in the production of the hospital social order. This is in line with the cognitive turn in contemporary social theory and in particular the new institutionalism (Power and DiMaggio, 1991: 22). In the first part of this section we examine the interlinkage between professional identity and normative or value commitments, cognitive mechanisms, and the construction of hospital order. A later part of this section explores certain limits of cognitive and organisational stabilisation, in particular the role of power and social change factors in de-stabilisation.

Cognitive Balancing Processes and the Hospital Order

As pointed out in Chapter 7, medical personnel experience considerable cognitive imbalance and associated tensions in the care and maintenance of braindead donors and organ harvesting. Dissonant communications, actions, and experiences arise because the actors participating in a hospital order do not have complete control over events, developments, communications, etc. They must interact with "outsiders" (namely, patients, next-of-kin), who may not understand and may question or challenge the patterns of the hospital order, the medical perspective, authority relationships, and cognitive and judgement processes. Moreover, even among medical personnel, deviance may occur because of mistakes, miscalculations, the pressure of contradictory demands, substantial changes in their action settings (through, for example, the introduction of new technologies, techniques, or other innovations).

Also, in section above was discussed how hospitals, as other organisations, operate to establish and maintain a stable cognitive and normative order. This is accomplished in part through various practices that deal with or resolve cognitive imbalance or dissonance in connection with key features, events and development of the hospital order. Institutionalised rituals and discourses resolve or neutralise cognitive imbalance by discounting, re-interpreting, or redefining the incongruent or dissonant cognitions, actions, or experiences – thereby preserving particular cognitions, judgements and actions derived from and legitimised by the social order of the hospital (such practices contribute, in part, to maintaining the boundary between the hospital ward(s) and the outside world (Anspach, 1993:163). That is, a key problem is to *maintain a stable judgement or cognition in the face of contradictory information, cognitions, and experiences.* Those faced with contradictory experiences or information *have responsibility for their judgements and actions (or those of others) but lack complete information and control. Thus, not only are these situations of uncertainty but of danger and risk* (Machado, 1990).

In the flux and flow of any action situation, there are events, processes, and developments that cannot be completely controlled. Information is ambiguous or contradictory. Actors may experience cognitive imbalance and dissonance in the situation. In some cases, the problems arise due to variation in situation, judgement, and action. In other cases, exogenous events and developments lead to dissonance and imbalance. These problems are often minimised within organisations where a high degree of routinisation and standardisation are achieved – that is, the situations can be highly structured and regulated ("tight-coupling" in Perrow (1979)). But, as much organisational research has shown, there are often situations where there is considerable "task uncertainty" or "environmental turbulence" (Burns and Stalker, 1961; Perrow, 1979; Scott, 1981). In our view, it is precisely these conditions which generate situations of cognitive ambiguity and imbalance. Such cognitive processes – and the connection to balance theory – have not been stressed in the organisational literature (concerning such problems as those of ambiguity and uncertainty see, however, Burns and Stalker (1961), Perrow (1979), March and Olsen(1976)).

What has been of particular interest to the research are the organisational processes of information selectivity, re-interpretation and re-framing that operate to stabilise cognitions. There is "organisational bias": a focus on and selectivity of particular data, events, and developments; and a disregard or blindness to other data, events, and developments. Organisational rituals play an important role in defining situations (in some instances, contrary to data or experience), thereby providing a particular experience or sense of the situation, and stabilising the situation. Information and accounting systems, which provide the bases for many organisational discourses, operate selectively to facilitate or maintain a certain cognitive stability and social order. Routinised reporting – and accounting – serve to stabilise core cognitions, beliefs, and judgements of the organisational order. In addition to formalised arrangements that resolve or reduce imbalance, there are also typically informal processes, for example that subordinates or colleagues simply do not report certain events, conditions, or developments, so that many situations of imbalance remain hidden or unattended to.

Many of the core cognitive elements, decisions, and actions which have been the focus here are organisational, not individual, in character. OTC treats cognitions, judgements, decisions, and particular actions not as individual undertakings, but as institutional, structural, interactional. It stresses the relevance to organisational analysis of understanding cognitive processes such as the generation of cognitive imbalance and balancing mechanisms. In particular, it addresses experiences and processes of cognitive imbalance that arise in relation to beliefs, classifications, representations, decisions, or other cognitions associated with core elements of an organisation, those elements that are closely linked to identity, legitimacy, authority, status. In the case of a hospital order, identity is closely associated with its key professional groups, physicians, surgeons, nurses. The latter are responsible – and feel themselves responsible – and vigorously defend the core elements of the hospital medical order, and cognitions, judgements, and acts associated with or representing that order. They represent the organisation in a certain sense. "Self" or identity is connected to these components – and to cognitive elements based on or derived from these. Cognitive as well as social order are maintained in part through particular organisational practices such as institutionalised rituals and discourses.

One key notion emerging from this theoretical formulation is the linkage between cognitive processes and social order, and the importance of *cognitive stabilisation* within the hospital order. This is especially so since two key features of the order, its authority and legitimacy, are closely associated with its particular judgement frame: medical science and the service dedication of health care professionals. This frame provides a common knowledge and normative orientation for members of the organisation.[187] It orients actors. It includes classification schemes that are the basis for distinguishing, describing and analysing the problems of their clients, the ways in which these problems are to be analysed, dealt with, or solved. (The more formal, systematic forms of such knowledge schemes are found in science, appearing as typologies, models, generalisations, laws, etc.) The frame also provides particular conceptions and normative guidelines for social relationships and organisation. Important distinctions are made and shape the ways that actors in the hospital order view their situations, think about them, act in them.

In the OTC perspective the shared judgement frame (a particular normative-cognitive structure) is the collective basis for actors to define, classify, and judge situations, events, actions, persons, problems, and the solutions of problems, and to produce a particular social order. Actors in some positions, for example physicians vis-à-vis the nursing staff, have greater responsibility and authority to define, classify, and judge than others (the characteristic features of this domination relationship, entailing a gender aspect as well, cannot be examined in this context). The shared frame enables members of the collective to organise and co-ordinate their activities – and to exercise stabilising controls that contribute in many instances to maintaining the order in face of disturbances, challenges, and even crisis. It is the basis for them to collectively regulate not only themselves and one another but to deal with or manage outsiders. This capacity, demonstrated in day-to-day activities, reinforces their commitments and loyalties to the normative and knowledge bases, since participants can trust, or have confidence that the social order will work more or less effectively and that it will command authority, legitimacy, and loyalty and respect from others, other things being equal.

A variety of control mechanisms are used to regulate, neutralise, offset, or avoid cognitive disturbances, ambiguities, dissonance, and so forth. Social regulation and stabilisation takes place in part through obvious sanctioning and social control processes, which are visible within most types of organisations. The OTC emphasises combinations of cognitive and interaction processes (e.g. rituals and discourses) that contribute to the maintenance and stabilisation of social order. Social controls are exercised over outsiders with whom the organisation (or its representatives) must deal, both in acquiring resources, technologies, and expertise, but also in dealing with their clients (and their next-of-kin). There are risks, and a certain vulnerability, involved in dealing with outsiders, particularly the outsiders defined as their clients, namely the supposed beneficiaries of the order. The latter may make excessive or unpredictable demands, and act in ways which disrupt the order, in part by mobilising other outsiders, such as the mass media, authorities including courts. Thus, while some social controls such as economic and administrative sanctions are important factors in hospital regulation, many disturbances and problems of stabilisation cannot be handled simply by such obvious social controls, although these play a significant role. Considerable social regulation, stabilisation, and maintenance occur through collective communicative actions and other symbolic actions and interactions. Here we stress rituals and discourses in regulative and stabilisation processes; these contribute to maintaining and stabilising not only particular cognitive elements, but also commitments to core values and the medical judgement frame of the hospital order.

Limits of Cognitive Stabilisation

The Reality and Power Principles. The cognitive stabilising mechanisms – underlying dissonance reduction – operate in a purely constructive way, that is beyond "reality controls or constraints". There are many historical examples of "blindness" to information, facts, and messages, for instance about increasing perils or pending catastrophes (the "Titanic syndrome"?). However, in general, there are limits to the extent to which actors through their discourses, rituals, and organisational procedures, can reduce or eliminate dissonance. Rituals may minimise or reduce dissonance highlighting certain aspects of a situation (and downplaying other), and/or in re-interpreting information stabilise cognitions in the immediate situation. However, in the longer-run, the "world talks back", "imposes itself". There are other authoritative (or powerful) agents who have a say about defining reality or determining what is the right or appropriate cognition, judgement, or action in a given situation, or what information is appropriate or to be selected and attended to, what are valid interpretations, what is relevant or irrelevant; what discourses and rituals are appropriate or not to the situation. *These and related matters may become matters of contestation and conflict, challenging what otherwise had been a stable judgement frame and interaction order.* For instance, the doctor in charge or the team has judged the patient as "dead", but outside authorities might investigate and consider contrary evidence. The group's own discourse – and normative accounting – is not exclusively authoritative or decisive.

The dissonant or ambiguous information may come from a very concrete experience or from an authoritative source (for instance, one having considerable legitimacy), and, therefore, cannot be easily denied, selected away or simply re-interpreted. In the latter case, the dissonant data or communications are backed by persons with the authority or power to compel an accounting, or accountability of the actors involved! For instance, another unit of the organisation responsible for checking and controlling judgements and procedures may introduce or validate contradictory information or interpretations. Or an entirely external unit or organisation may do this. Hence, it is important that those within the organisation responsible and accountable for judgements make use of the same information, and follow established (or "right and proper") procedures for making judgements and acting on the basis of the information. Their cognitive processes and discourses – at least as publicly formulated – are required to correspond to or fit with those of the superordinate or more encompassing system.

Social Change and Increases in Cognitive Instability. Innovation in techniques and technologies sets the stage for new problems and predicaments and the de-stabilisation of established judgement frames or cognitive configurations. Consider, for example, the new definition of death, which is more technically demanding (a particular medical competence is required). It leaves some of the personnel, who lack competence, uncertain. Even when patients are defined as dead, they may not differ in appearance from persons in a coma. This is a new type of situation, generating new problems of dissonance. The situation is characterised by multiple meanings, or unclarity. "What's going on here" in the context of brain death is not supposed to be vague or unclear.[188] Quite the contrary, death by neurological criteria is most often legally defined, as well as the procedures for its determination ascertained by means of well-established clinical or mechanical tests.

Major technical and technological innovations lead to conditions, events, patterns which do not fully fit actors' established ways of categorising, perceiving, assessing the situation, and acting. The changes are of enough import to weaken the "taken for granted" nature of a previous frame of rules and practices. Actors are confronted with new problem situations, patterns of action, and a repertoire of solutions to problems which do not fit with the judgement frame (with particular classification schemes, collective representations, organising principles and rules) they have employed thus far. This sets the stage for increased or new types of dissonance as well as the greater likelihood of dissonance experiences.

In particular, organ transplantation disrupts rituals and discourses relating to life and death. It raises new ethical   dilemmas and predicaments.

(1) For instance, the introduction of procedures to keep a dead patient "functioning" until the organs can be removed leads to ambiguous and dissonant situations discussed earlier.

(2) In general, there are continual pressures to act more efficiently, for instance to eliminate or to minimise "delays". The timing and arrangements for organ procurement often take precedent over the needs or feelings of the next-of-kin. Even if they have an opportunity to be present with the dying patient, this time must be organised, controlled and regulated. Medical personnel have to prepare the skin and make sterile draping for procurement surgery (here Fox (1993:233) refers to the transfer of dying but not yet dead patients to the operating room).

Organ transplantation has operated in such a way as to mix up or confuse expectations of personnel and next-of-kin: on the one hand, to procure (and preserve) organs and, on the other, to give consolation and to make the situation as pleasant as possible for next-of-kin. It functions best if next-of-kin are not involved during the process. One nurse reported, "I have also seen next-of-kin fail to understand that the patient is dead but in some instances when the patient is taken to the operating room to remove organs they have asked if the patient will be 'well' after the operation".

In general, the problems of dissonance are particularly prominent under conditions of social or socio-technical change, for instance, when new techniques and technologies are introduced. The established routines, criteria for judgement, procedures, etc. no longer lead to the minimisation or reduction of dissonance, but rather to its intensification.

Of particular importance is the way in which innovations in techniques and technologies may not only disrupt established information and accounting systems but also discourses and rituals that earlier had contributed to effectively stabilising judgements and experiences relating to life and death matters. *That is, actors experience new types (or levels) of ambiguities and dissonance – or old ones – which can no longer be readily or systematically resolved or minimised through established organisational means.*

Discussion and Conclusions

The proposition that the resolution of cognitive imbalance and balancing processes are organisational phenomena, not simply individual experiences, distinguishes OTC from the classical social psychological balance theories. The approach, in line with the developments of the new institutionalism

(March and Olsen, 1984; Powell and DiMaggio, 1991, among others), establishes the centrality of cognitive processes in the study of organisational behaviour. It identifies a practical, non-calculative, non-rational side of organisational motivation and action, in part by emphasising the centrality of contradiction and cognitive disturbance in the context of a professional organisation, and in part by emphasising the moral or normative aspects in these processes, in particular those relating closely to self-conception and identity.

As stressed in the chapter, professional actors experience meaningful or salient inconsistency and contradiction – and balancing processes are activated – within particular judgement frames, that is, socially constructed cognitive-normative structures. Such frames are part of – are closely connected to – their collective self-conceptions or identities. Physicians and nurses as key professionals in hospital settings embody particular judgement frames and collective self-conceptions. Their identities commit them to – hold them responsible for – key cognitive and normative components of the judgement frame: that is, particular collective representations and classification schemes; particular beliefs, norms and values; particular roles, conceptions of authority and status relationships in the hospital or more generally medical context. Experiences, communications, performance results, or other forms of data, which contradict or are incongruent with one or more such components, or their derivatives, cause distress and evoke balancing processes. Through particular organisational and professional rituals, discourses, props, and other situational structures, hospital professionals define their commitment to and reinforcement of professional identity or selfhood as well as to particular values and norms, particular roles, authority and status relations. In this way, OTC *conceptualises the dynamic interlinkage between professional identity and normative or value commitments, cognitive mechanisms, and ritualistic and emotional solidarity in medical groups, and views these factors as central to the social construction of the hospital order.* Indeed, what has been of interest here are the particular types of contradiction and other sources of destabilisation, and the cognitive and related organisational mechanisms that resolve dissonance or imbalance and stabilise the social order.

OTC identifies major sources of cognitive contradiction and imbalance in the practical conditions and processes of professional organisations. It explains in part why medical professionals find some interactions, events, and developments more acceptable or "right" than others – or conversely some are more problematic and unacceptable than others. These assessments often have nothing directly to do with organisational goals, or matters of instrumental rationality. The theory also explains also why some routines such as particular organisational rituals and discourses are highly stable –

and repeatedly utilised – even if they are not "rationally" motivated. Indeed, in many instances the actors engaged in these processes are not aware of the function or role they play; they feel right to them, they are emotionally satisfying. Typically they are unable to explain why they feel distress or react emotionally to particular contradictions or cognitive disturbances, and not others. The theory provides some explanation of why certain instances of cognitive imbalance and dissonance evoke strong emotional, even passionate, responses: specifically in instances where collective identity – and representations and expressions of this identity in particular cognitions, actions and practices – are at stake or highly salient.

The theory identifies a number of organisational and professional processes and arrangements that operate to minimise cognitive imbalance and dissonance with respect to the social definition of the situation, strategic social facts, and the derivations from the judgement frame that agents utilise in their ongoing activities, judgements, decisions, etc. Cognitive imbalance is resolved through selection and denial, redefinition and re-framing, re-interpretation, and distortion. In other words, such processes serve to stabilise the cognitive field and the social order at the core of which are the *collective professional selves – and well as individual selves in given positions and roles in the organisation.*

Meanings are continually being produced through the organisational processes of dealing with anomalies and other deviations from the "normal" cognitive and social order. Not anyone can activate or participate in these mechanisms of normalisation. Only members, and typically only certain key members, have the authority to initiate or conduct a particular discourse or ritual, or to establish or make use of particular organisational props and arrangements. And this must be done not arbitrarily, but in particular ways consistent with professional conceptions and norms. More precisely, one cannot simply select away (or ignore) professionally highly salient information; or one cannot arbitrarily re-interpret, re-frame, or re-define realities. There are powerful and meaningful professional and hospital as well as legal norms constraining as well as facilitating framing, interpretative, and transformative possibilities.

Implications for Organisational Theory

The hospital is a professional organisation where authority and legitimacy – and other features of the social order – are based to a great extent on: (I) expert knowledge (medical science) rather than on legal correctness or economic power (although such legal and economic factors also enter in); (II) a value orientation toward serving the health and welfare of patients. Medical personnel and other participants in contact with patients and next-of-kin believe in, and express commitment to, medical science and a professional value orientation to clients. Professionals recruited to a hospital receive training and socialisation prior to coming and on-the-job; they are also certified as having acquired professional judgement frames and performance skills necessary to occupy positions and play the role of "physician" or "nurse", as the case may be. Professional socialisation also entails the acquisition of certain value orientations, norms, forms of discourse, and rituals.

Does OTC have more general applicability, and, if so, to what extent? I have suggested it does so, partly through generalising several of the arguments, partly by offering illustrations from other types of social organisation. However, a more systematic (if only preliminary) answer to the question is warranted.

All organisations have mechanisms to maintain social order, for instance explicit social controls, regulations, and sanctions. In this chapter I have stressed organisational order grounded, in large part, on organisational practices of discourse and ritual to stabilise particular salient cognitions and a professional judgement frame within representational and classificatory systems as well as value and normative orientations. The principle is simple: *events, communications and cognitive elements that confuse, erode, challenge, endanger the social order – or particularly cognitions, judgements, or actions which are closely associated with, or which are essential to constituting the order – become sources of tension and challenge, and subject to regulative and stabilising actions.* The problem of cognitive stabilisation and social order is common to all sustained collective activity and organisation, especially for the organisational elite or professionals who direct and manage the organisations: order can be accomplished through a variety of social controls. But some controls – or mechanisms of control – are more appropriate than others. Organisations differ, of course, in terms of their tasks and goals, their fundamental judgement frames, social representations and classification schemes, and normative bases.

Professional organisations oriented to clients have an obvious normative base – the value orientation to the welfare or good of their clients. They rely particularly on normative and persuasive rhetoric to deal with ambiguities and dissonance relating to core aspects of their social order. Their discourses refer to expert knowledge – or expert authority – and also make normative appeals relating to their mission of, for example, saving lives and healing the sick. Professional or scientific competence as well as consideration of clients' welfare are stressed, directly or indirectly, for these are the ultimate bases of authority and legitimacy. This gives professional, service-oriented organisations such as modern hospitals their identity. In such organisations, outsiders but also many members of the organisations must be assured that, for instance, there is less dissonance than otherwise might appear to be the case, that particular collective representations, judgements, decisions, or actions are right and proper, and derive from an application of expert knowledge in trying to improve or maintain clients' welfare.

Professional, service-oriented organisations cannot easily maintain social order merely through economic incentives, or coercion. Whenever ambiguities and dissonance arise, professional members communicate their commitment and loyalty to the judgement frame, authority structures, and the social order – through particular discourses and rituals. This is especially important in dealing with clients, or their relatives/friends, where the use of crude sanctions would be inappropriate, if not unethical, and in general, probably ineffective. These outsiders are to be persuaded, convinced of particular definitions of reality and attributions – but this cannot be accomplished through a long process of socialisation/education (there is not the time and resources for this; this is precisely the type of process that health care groups such as physicians and nurses undergo). Patients, their next-of-kin, and others must also be convinced or persuaded to fit into or accept the hospital order – and its implications. Hence, particular authoritative discourses, rituals, and other symbolic actions are utilised in defining or stabilising their cognitions – and, thereby, contributing to the maintenance of the social order.

In professional, service-oriented organisations, their cognitive processes are structured and stabilised through normative conviction and through the systematic application of a *particular judgement frame*, based on science and systematic knowledge, and collective processes such as rituals and discourses. While all modern organisations have to a greater extent expert knowledge and normative foundations, these are core features of professional, service oriented organisations such as health care facilities. The arrangements of other types of organisations (Etzioni, 1975) may be based largely on remuneration (for example, work places, whether private or public where people perform duties or functions, obey authority in exchange for wages and salaries) or on coercion (e.g. prisons and closed mental hospitals (Goffman, 1961)).

Therefore, it would appear that the scope of the theory developed here covers *professional, service-oriented organisations*, that is organisations with an expert knowledge base and a strong value commitment to clients. In such organisations, authority and status and the exercise of social control and influence within the organisations and in relation to other organisations and the larger society derive to a great extent from special expert knowledge and normative appeals and authority. In future work, we will apply the theory to investigating not only health care organisations other than hospitals, but also educational and scientific institutions as well as other professional organisations that are service-oriented (organisations of lawyers, government agencies, and some church organisations).

It may be possible to extend the theory presented here even to types of organisations other than professional, service-oriented ones, to the extent that these have a strong self-conception image and identity, a normative base to which members are deeply committed at the same time as they must deal with outsiders and events that disturb, disrupt, challenge, and destabilise the particular organisational order where key mechanisms for stabilising and maintaining the order take place through normative appeals and references to specialised expert knowledge. In other words, it would seem an obvious extension of OTC to explore its relevance to normatively oriented organisations in general (Etzioni, 1975).

These mechanisms may also be widespread in other types of organisations, although their forms may vary considerably.

(1) In a rigid, administrative system, the leadership or elite may believe deeply that they or their policies and strategies will succeed in achieving organisational goals. Such hope is often maintained through a number of dissonance reducing mechanisms, that is through particular processes of organisational selectivity, re-definition and re-interpretation as stabilising processes. Those subordinates who deliver messages or information that would contradict the elite's judgement and horizon of hope may be *sanctioned* severely and therefore avoid delivering such contradictory messages (in oppressive systems heavy sanctions may include execution).[189] Thus, subordinates may positively re-interpret information and systematically conceal information from their superiors. *This contributes of course to the stabilisation of the elite's judgement frame* and their underlying beliefs and horizon of hope. Many rank-and-file members may have no strong commitment to the truth or to the long-term status, authority, or legitimacy of the order, and, therefore, experience no major qualms about going along with the illusion – often this is because their self-conceptions are not closely identified with the organisation or its management. It's ultimate success or failure is not *their* success or failure. Consequently, any challenge to the perspective and judgements of the organisational elite may have to come *from outside the organisation*, in the form of powerful agents or forces (market or electoral forces), that cannot be ignored or denied. Of course, rebels may emerge within the organisation – offering a different vision of reality, and struggling with the elite, possibly gaining allies from agents outside the organisation as well as from within the elite

itself. But this presupposes a relatively open organisation, possibly with considerable security of tenure for employees.

(2) Expert authority and even charisma may be a basis for professional and administrative domination. We have seen this in the hospital context in the readiness of nurses and next-of-kin to accept in many instances the judgements of physicians and derivations of the medical judgement frame.[190] These patterns of acceptance serve to reinforce the social order. It reduces complexity and instability, as suggested earlier. This same type of mechanism can operate in other authoritative settings.

(3) In a more, open egalitarian organisation or group, commitment to particular judgements and their stabilisation depend on establishing and maintaining consensus on the basis of judgements derived from a common judgement frame. In religious groups, this is their religious frame of reference. Among physicians, this is accomplished in part by making use of objective means of defining reality, selecting data, etc. as well as through the utilisation of particular discourses. Among physicians, the commitment to and homage to the *scientific judgement frame* – together with the techniques, technologies, and discourses appropriate for medical settings – operate to stabilise on a collective level particular cognitions, judgements, and commitments. In all egalitarian groups and organisations, collective discourses and rituals such as discussed and analysed in the chapter are a common denominator – although the forms, language, and symbolism will differ.

(4) As suggested above, there are likely to be limits to how far a group may go in shaping and maintaining its horizon of hope, its faith, its judgement frame, its beliefs, judgements, and commitments – above all when the organisation or group must deal with *outside forces and agents*, which confront core groups of the organisation with events, conditions, developments that contradict their judgement frame, or its particular derived cognitions, judgements, and actions based on it.[191] Organisations or groups which dominate their immediate surroundings or internal environment, as in (1) above, may reconstruct reality successfully for long periods. Ultimately, however, there is always the risk that the real world comes "crashing down on them".

Instrumental Rationality and Organisational Order

Most modern formal organisations structure and activities that are, at least in principle, intended to accomplish given goals in a more or less rational manner (Blau and Scott, 1962; Burns and Flam, 1987; Scott, 1981).[192] However, OTC implies that several *key organisational features, arrangements, and processes are designed and evolve in order to deal with cognitive imbalance or dissonance and subsequent distress and disorder.* Cognitive balancing or stabilisation processes may contribute to the maintenance of incorrect as well as correct beliefs or judgements. That is, a new truth may be denied (as in science, it may be difficult to judge whether anomalies with respect to an established paradigm are to be explained away, or seen as secondary, or to serve as a point of departure for developing a new paradigm). Thus, OTC implies that there is more to organisational behaviour than striving for or achieving explicit goals effectively and efficiently. Organisational members, in particular professional groups, act in ways to maintain cognitive order and stability, and this is closely connected with a particular conception or definition of themselves and the hospital order in which they play central roles. Information selectivity and denial, re-definition and re-interpretation of situations, definition of particular situations, events, and developments as non-relevant are everyday processes in organisations. Such processes may lead to "non-rational", "counter-productive", or "ineffective" organisational performances. But such non-rational patterns are explained in OTC, not as the result of human irrationality or folly, but in terms of the stabilisation of cognition, and social order.

(1) In a certain sense, organisational and professional rituals and discourses as well as organisational features and props protect key groups against the full impact of multiple and potentially contradictory and destabilising messages (including "truthful" but disconcerting information). At the same time, these stabilising mechanisms serve to balance cognitions and judgement frames and maintain social order, they entail to a greater or lesser extent a certain denial or distortion of important data and information. In this way, serious problems – even potentially catastrophic problems – may be ignored or defined as non-serious. OTC brings our attention then to the fact that professional groups and organisations often insulate themselves from disruptive or disturbing pieces of information, experiences, and communications. And while the group and organisational mechanisms identified by the theory play a key role in cognitive and emotional solidarity and in the maintenance of the hospital social order, they also entail bias, distortion, half-truths, illusions, blindness, and rationalisations (Goffman, 1967:43). That such factors play a major part in integrating a group or moral community is a basic insight, if not a principle of general sociology. Such factors are particularly interesting, as we have suggested here, when they operate among professionals oriented to empirical science, "truth", and rationality. All moral communities share in common that they are held together – and social order maintained – through cognitive balancing mechanisms, grounded in rituals, special discourses, props, and

situational structures within groups and organisations. There is a continual production of meaning and also bias and distortion. In this sense, many medical as well as scientific discourses, rituals and props can be – and are – used in magical or mythical ways (Elias, 1996).

(2) The theory outlined here states that "rational" judgmental processes and "irrational" cognitive balance processes are not opposing or alternative conceptualisations. On the contrary, they are both characteristic and essential features of human practical action. Ironically, non-rational cognitive processes and discourses as well as various organisational or inter-organisational rituals contribute to stabilising judgement frameworks (and a social order) which are ostensibly "rational". *Cognitive balancing processes – no matter how irrational – provide a collective frame which enable actors, in our study here physicians and nurses, to make rational type decisions (in part, making use of science and modern technologies) in pursuit of organisational goals.*

9 Medicine and Legal Regulation

Legal Regulation of Transplantation: The Swedish Transplant Acts

The expansion of many biotechnical tools in medical therapy and research requires a substantial supply of human biological material. Blood, for example, is a vital element in surgical procedures. Governments, policy makers, and international organisations respond to these developments by formulating laws and guidelines to regulate, for example, organ and tissue extraction and use.

Until 1988 medical authorities in Sweden had potential control rights over a person's body parts unless the person had expressed opposition to organ extraction, that is the principle of presumed consent (see Chapter 3). The revised Transplant Law (1987), applied between 1988 and 1996, was designed to protect in large part the bodily integrity and autonomy of the individual citizen, for instance preventing body parts being taken against her will. The 1987 Act allowed "minor body parts"[193] to be extracted from a deceased without prior consent or authorisation of relatives. Also, residuals from surgery could be used by the hospital, although in principle the person was supposed to be informed of any intent to use the material. This included foetal tissue (which has been increasingly used for research as well as therapeutic purposes), but a request for authorisation from the mother is a common procedure in this case. In general, hospitals in Sweden take residuals and smaller parts, whether from living or dead persons. The value of the "common good" was prioritised when it came to deceased persons and minor amounts of biological material. Rights over body parts and corpses have shifted in the past 40 years (since the 1958 Act on the Use of Tissue and Other Biological Material). With the amendment to the Transplants Act, from 1 January 1996, Sweden returned to the condition prior to 1988 of presumed consent.

In general, the body (of a human subject or citizen) is a space where a matrix of rights and rules define and regulate the individual's and others' relationships to her body. The law makes important distinctions in the demand for consent for medical bodily actions, taking into consideration the degree of invasiveness of the medical procedure. This general principle (see Rynning, 1994) was apparently applied in creating a division between the consent requirements for "minor" and "major" body parts, in the Transplants Act of 1975. The rationale of such a principle is understandable, but, with regard to more recent medical procedures (e.g. genetic manipulation), rather outdated.

The person's "body" is more than an anatomical or physiological entity attached to the person. It is also a social construction that in part is fashioned in the legal discourse. There is no explicit concept of "body" in the legislation. The underlying assumptions about bodies are not especially clear. However, a body can be understood as a legally defined space or domain of the individual person. It is understood that the body is not an object that the individual person can sell, destroy or give away in a testament (donations to museums and medical institutions as recipients are excepted).[194] In short it is not simply property. This notion of "the body" rests on contemporary western conceptions such as the Cartesian duality of body and thought as one of the philosophical bases of the concept of "rational man". This basically means that man (rationality) is opposed to nature (body). For instance, if the body is seen as an aspect or expression of the soul, then conceptions of bodies, and values attached to them, will differ substantially from conceptions that separate body and soul, where the latter is considered the truly human (and rational) part.

Persons have also been differentiated in the Transplant laws on the basis of their status or level of rational agency, that is their capacity to reason and decide rationally and, therefore, stand accountable for their actions.[195] Thus, the agency of persons who were defined as mentally disabled or incompetent was not applicable to decision-making over their body parts, e.g. in making living donations. Children's agency is not fully applicable to their body parts (their bodies are legally under the agency or control of their authorities). In general, not everybody is defined equally before the law, at least in the area of organ donation.

Law and Medicine in the Regulation of Medical Action on Bodies

Through investigations covering also other laws regulating medical actions on the body, I found that the laws not only concern particular actions on the body and the use of the body and body parts in clinical medicine and research, but also legally sanctioned *definitions of the person and her body and the distribution of rights over the body and body parts*, matters that will be explored below. These explore a few aspects of the complex interplay between medicine and law, focusing on a complex of laws, including transplant Acts, regulating medical intervention on bodies. Among the Acts considered are those regulating autopsy, abortion, fertilisation, use of foetal tissue and medical residuals, and transplantation. These define, divide up, and construct through legal discourses, a body whose boundaries and internal relations do not correspond with common everyday notions of biological bodies. They define a set of relationships linking social agents, including the person herself, to her body. The study identifies the agents who have the right to decide over various types of treatment and uses of the body and body parts. Several of the key dimensions patterning the distribution of such rights over the body are: the legally defined level of reason or rationality of the individual (her capability to decide for herself), the degree of invasiveness of the action, the relative value or weight given to individual bodily integrity and competing values relating to "public interest" or the collective good. These laws, among other things, define the reasonable or rational individual who may decide over her body and they determine the mix between the autonomy of the individual and her body and the "public interest" or common good in controlling the body and body parts.

In my approach laws are seen to encode, often implicitly, sociocultural assumptions, concepts, beliefs, and values concerning, for example, human rationality, the nature of the citizen's body, and donation or giving of the body and body parts. The laws also define and construct new conceptions and meanings of the relation of the person and her body to the state, as well as to other social agents. Thus, laws can be investigated as the bases for the construction of different "legally constituted bodies" where, for instance, access to (and uses of) certain parts of the body are legally sanctioned while others are excluded. The laws also encode a particular conception of the reasonable or "rational" individual who can decide over her body and also others defined as lacking this competence (for example, very young children, the senile, other mentally incompetent or ill persons as well as persons temporarily unconscious, sedated, or under the influence of alcohol or narcotic). In the case of the Transplant Acts (Machado, 1996b), one can identify legally sanctioned forms of, and assumptions about, giving, specifically the giving of body parts defined as organ or "tissue donation". Moreover, this legislation not only regulates and legitimises practices that make use of the body and body parts in clinical medicine and research, but also engenders legally sanctioned definitions of individual rights and autonomy. Some of these definitions and their implications for the construction of the "social self" are examined, e.g. the character and distribution of rights over the body and its parts.

Such socio-legal studies (Machado, 1996a, 1996b) treat laws and regulations as cultural artefacts, investigating how they define, and operate as a symbol of, what is regarded as normalising and objective, encoding sociocultural assumptions, concepts, and values. Law also functions as a powerful normative guide in defining and constructing social reality, in particular the citizen's "body", in part conceptualised within a space of rights delineated in medical laws.

Legal Discourses and Bodies

It is no longer controversial to state that the "person" is socially constituted or that such a concept is social in nature and rooted in particular historical and social geographical (Western) circumstances. Bodies are another matter, they are often regarded as natural (non-social) entities or facts. However, contemporary sociological research suggests otherwise (see Featherstone et al., 1991; Turner, 1984, 1992). It follows that conceptions of the "body" are relative not only to historical or particular cultural circumstances but also relative to epistemological preferences.[196] In this sense bodies, subject to contextual definitions, are socially constituted. *In modern society, one of the important domains where this constitution takes place is in legal discourse.* Thus, the study of the law as discourse is not limited to specific laws or to the activity of litigation or litigators; rather it is the study of these laws as they operate as symbols for what is legal, honourable, natural and objective (Eisenstein, 1988).

Moreover, not every conception of "body" is equally central. Some conceptions (e.g. those legally sanctioned) are defined as more central than others and enjoy dominance.[197] An illustration of this is the legally sanctioned conception of a body as dead following irreversible brain failure. Here, the shift of theories/praxis in medical science about death-life boundaries is institutionalised and endorsed by the law: a non-functioning brain replaces the absence of breath and heart beating as a sign of death.

What do laws reveal about cultural assumptions, conceptions, values, norms in a society? For example, what do they reveal about the assumptions of "individual agency", or about social relationships (between, for example, state and individual), or the organisation of society; or about desirable and undesirable social states. The method is to select a set of laws relating to an area such as "treatment of the body", for instance the Acts regulating organ extraction. Typically, the various laws define a set of relationships linking social agents, including the person herself, to the body; defining, for instance, which agents have the right to decide over treatment and use of the body or body parts, and under what conditions.

Rights and Constraints with Respect to Medical Actions on Bodies

The person's bodily integrity, in Sweden, is stipulated in the Constitution. It is protected by general administrative laws regulating general medical procedures, by specific laws overseeing particular medical actions, and by sanctions in the Criminal Code. According to the Constitution, fully competent adults have rights to bodily integrity. All citizens are protected from coercive bodily procedures (e.g. torture, capital punishment) but also from medical actions such as physical tests, surgical operations, and similar procedures carried out on a person without her authorisation (Proposition 1975/76:290).[198] It is also stated that any coercive action overriding a person's basic rights has to be supported by her consent, by another law[199] or by a state of emergency. In principle, a person has to give consent to any bodily procedures performed on her; otherwise such an action carried out on her body against her will is a legal transgression. Nonetheless, medical procedures, more than any other actions on persons' bodies, are released from strict demands of consent (Jareborg in Rynning, 1994:432-433).[200] Moreover, it is in the domain of Public Administrative Law that the legal dimension of private persons' bodies is delineated.

The Health Care Act (Law, 1928:763) is the widest and more encompassing Swedish law concerning medical procedures. This Act has the character of a legal frame (*ramlag*) more than of a detailed regulation of medical procedures. Medical laws that regulate particular medical procedures are the Abortion Act (Law, 1974:595); the Sterilisation Act (Law, 1975:580); the Insemination Act (Law, 1984:1140-FB); the Act About Fertilisation Outside the Body (Law, 1988:711- SFS); the Act about Forensic Psychiatric Care (Law, 1991:1129-LTP); the Act on the Prevention of (spreading of) Infectious Diseases (Law, 1988:1472) and the Transplants Act (Law, 1995:831), as it relates to living persons. Regarding deceased persons, important laws are the Criteria for Determination of a Person's Death, the Transplants Act (Law, 1995:831), the Autopsy Act (Law, 1975:191) and other subsidiary regulations.

Modern law (mainly through state agency) defines the positions (rights, duties, and responsibilities) of distinct categories of actors in relation to the individual body in medical procedures. The main actors considered and thus defined by these regulations are the individual person herself as citizen,[201] relevant authorities[202] (including in this case the hospital authority, the collective [*allmänna*], the government [*statsmakt*],the physician responsible for the patient). Others may be women, minors, those defined as mentally incompetent or senile, drug addicts, alcoholics, adults with dangerous transmissible diseases, the mature foetus, next-of-kin, and guardians.

In this way, it is possible to map out a set of social relationships in terms of a matrix of rights, possibilities, and obligations associated with a person's body as specified in laws regarding medical actions. The following rights are of interest: the right to receive or refuse medical treatment; the right to decide if a part of one's body can be removed (donation, etc.); the right to determine what is done with one's body after death, including possible removal of parts; the right to decide how any part removed is to be used, who is to receive it, etc. Besides addressing such questions, I explore ways in which certain legal and medical distinctions play a part in the articulation of the matrix of rights, for example the distinction between major and minor medical actions (and body parts), between living and dead bodies, and between persons who are defined as mentally competent and those who are not. Thus, important distinctions in the analysis are concerned with the type and status of agents involved (state agents, professionals, patients, next-of-kin, or others) and the various types of action. The rights of different categories of actors in relation to medical actions on bodies will be presented below.

Distribution of Bodily Rights

Several of the key dimensions patterning the distribution of individual bodily rights in medical procedures are: societal values concerning individual integrity as opposed to the common good; level of rationality of the individual; the impact[203] of the medical action on the body. Other dimensions that play a role in the allocation of bodily rights are age,[204] sex, civil state, and nationality of the subject. These dimensions reflect cultural values encoded to a greater or lesser extent in the legal system.[205] The laws constitute matrices of rights defining and regulating who has *the right to decide over treatment and use of the body or body parts as a function of the legal status of the person.* Table 11 presents several key medical actions varying in terms of *the invasiveness of the actions* (rows I., II.), *actions relating to reproductive function* (rows II., IV., V.), *the use of body parts for living and necrotransplantation* (rows VI., VII., VIII.), *autopsy* (row IX.), and *dissection* (row X.).

1. The personal and bodily integrity of the individual citizen is implicitly or explicitly applied in constitutional principles and multiple laws. These basic principles come into play in the formulation of new laws and the rewriting of old laws but can be restricted in their application for reason of limited rationality of the person or the common good. The law

Table 11. Status of the person and the right to determine medical actions (1996)

	STATUS OF THE PERSON				
MEDICAL ACTIONS ON BODIES	Normal citizen	Non-conscious patients	Children, mentally handicapped	Mentally ill, senile	Dead
I. Invasive medical actions in hospitals	full individual right	public right (physician and relatives)	limited right (shared with custodian)	limited right (with custodian)	to allow survival of the foetus
II. Tests and non-invasive medical actions in hospitals	full individual right, often tacit consent	public right (physician)	limited right (shared with custodian)	limited right (shared with custodian)	public right if organ donation
III. Abortion	full right up to 18th week pregnancy	•	full right up to 18th week *	full right up to 18th week *	•
IV. Insemination, in-vitro fertilisation	limited right (shared with husband)	•	•	•	•
V. Castration/ sterilisation	limited right (if not medically justified)	•	public/ limited right	public right	•
VI. Organ extraction from living donors	full individual right	•	limited right (custodian)	limited right (custodian)	•
VII. Organ extraction from cadaver donors	veto right	•	•	•	next-of-kin right
VIII. Tissue extraction from cadaver donors	public right	public right	public right	public right	public right
IX. Autopsy	•	•	•	•	limited right if forensic
X. Dissection	•	•	•	•	full individual right

* As long as she is mentally competent to understand the consequences of the procedure.

stresses that otherwise the mentally capable individual has full freedom to make decisions on the basis of her own judgement about measures to prevent or cure illness (Sjölenius 1989:59). The physician is supposed to be the patient's expert advisor and to accept the latter's decision. That is, an individual has the right to decide over her body (and larger) body parts. While legal experts play a major role in this, there is also a general acceptance of the ideology of individual citizen rights in a modern society such as Sweden. Medical and other professional interests involved in the medical treatment of bodies recognise and largely accept this.[206]

2. Persons as patients are entitled to receive health care, but this should be their decision. That is, no physician can, *in principle*, apply a treatment without the patient's approval. However, this is not a strict demand, since explicit consent for common medical procedures is not stated in the law (e.g. the Health Care Act), and is understood to be of a general kind.[207] This is indirectly formulated as the obligation of the health care personnel to give information, consultation and respect, with the latter as the only unrestricted demand.

3. The more consequential the intervention for the individual, that is, the more invasive the procedure, the more regulated and restrictive the control over medical action. The need to protect the person is recognised to a greater extent, for example, in regard to the removal of major unpaired organs from a living person (as opposed to hair, fingernails, etc.). However exceptions are made in two general types of cases: mental incapacity of the person and public interest in the medical action (even when minor actions are at stake). These are discussed in more detail below.

4. There are more severe restrictions on what a rational person can decide for herself when the law operates to assure protection of integrity (of autonomy) even at the expense of consent. Thus, the law prevents someone from donating her heart while alive. (This would be considered irrational or a form of "madness".) Although the law excludes this possibility, there is no law in Sweden against suicide. Nonetheless, one may be confined in a mental hospital "for one's own protection", even if there is no law against suicide or harming/maiming oneself.[208]

In the case that a person is considered a threat to public health and/or safety, the rights of the person to decide, even if fully competent, may be overridden and her freedom can be temporarily restricted. No medical treatment can be forced, however, on a person of "sound mind" – that is, as long as she is not defined as mentally ill – even if she suffers from a dangerous communicable disease.

5. Several medical actions are regarded as special, since they are the object of particular regulations, for example abortion and transplantation. These special medical actions on bodies require strict consent. Organ donation by mentally competent living donors is one. It is important to remark that this medical action *does not concern patients*. Another situation that does not concern patients is the Autopsy Act, where the individual integrity often recedes in the face of societal interests or needs (see below).

Special procedures concerned with the permanent suppression of reproductive functions such as sterilisation, castration and change of sex, also call for strict regulation. Social values regarding the importance of gender and reproduction in the formation of identity seem to play an important role in the very strict demands for protection. Concerning these procedures, persons above 18 but less than 23 (25 for castration), do not have full personhood, but are technically still considered minors.

6. Gender and reproduction are a special case in the law. Women are in principle full legal subjects, enjoying the same rights as men in the law. However, women appear to have a particular status in the law with respect to reproduction matters. For example, the Abortion Act concedes women the inalienable right to obtain an abortion *independently of their age*, up to 12 weeks of pregnancy. That is, the distinction between minors and adults is erased. The right to obtain an abortion is considerably safeguarded in the legislation. A women in the first trimester of pregnancy may herself decide on abortion. The foetus is treated in practice as a part of her body. In the second trimester, the consent of the hospital is required, and in the third, the hospital and the National Board of Health must approve the abortion. An interesting feature of this medical action is that age, and to a certain extent mental competence, do not enter in. Otherwise, adult women have restricted rights in all the other instances that concern reproductive issues. That is women's rights with respect to their bodies are very much determined by their reproductive capacities, since the right of the future child to live, to have a father, and eventually to know the identity of their genitor, are also protected. A woman shares her right to receive medical assistance to procreate with her husband or cohabitant (e.g. in the case of insemination, in-vitro fertilisation). The legal treatment of the particular matters of reproduction and sex, including also those individuals who choose to renounce their reproductive capacity, and those who choose to reverse their biological sex (e.g. transsexuals, homosexuals), is not fully consistent with and challenges the notion of a "gender-free citizen".

7. Next-of-kin includes spouse or cohabitant (*sammanboende*), children, parents and siblings. Homosexual relations are also taken into account

(Sjölenius, 1991).[209] Otherwise it is   a normal hospital practice to ask patients at the moment of their registration into a hospital which person should be contacted in case of need or emergency (patients have the right to refuse answering, and this should be respected except if they are seriously ill).[210] If this is the case, and the patient is unable to give consent to a treatment, the next-of-kin has to be informed.[211]

The role of the next-of-kin is a double one. They can act as information channels about their relative (information that may be relevant for the treatment) or as agents of the patient. Parents or legal custodians have the right to decide about minors or disabled by virtue of their responsibility for their safety and well-being, but the opinion of a minor is still to be considered.[212] The physician has the obligation of taking contact with the person or persons responsible for the minor. The older the minor, the more say she has about any procedures carried out on herself.[213] If parents or guardians consider the possibility of a minor or mentally disabled person in their charge as organ donors, authorisation of the Board of Health is required (and given only if exceptional reasons justify it, and if the donor agrees).

In the case of deceased donors, even if the decision or wishes of the individual are stressed, the family retains a residual role – for instance in Transplants and Autopsy Acts. In practice, the opinions and wishes of the family are taken into account (physicians tend to respect any eventual donation refusal of the next-of-kin even if the deceased would have expressed a positive wish to donate).

8. The relationship person-body is in principle broken when the person is declared dead. The body, now redefined as corpse, are the remains of the person. The regulations concerning corpses acknowledge the separation between body and person as complete. A law requires that corpses should be treated in accordance with the expected moral standards of the society, but not for reasons of their (residual) agency. "The regulation does not aim to protect the deceased and her relatives, but to protect the community against actions opposed to customary order" (my translation) (SOU:1989:98: 70).

A corpse is an entity of a very special kind. When a person dies, her status changes dramatically. Legally it is no longer a subject of right (and her property is distributed according to testamentary regulations). But the corpse does not qualify as an object of right either.[214] Legally, a person cannot give her corpse in testament, e.g. to her relatives, because a corpse cannot be the property of anybody. Nevertheless, a corpse can be given in testament to medical institutions for purposes of research and education. When grants of bodies or parts to museums and medicine schools are made, they are neither transfers of "property" nor "gifts". A person leaves her body for medical research or training in a "quasi-testamentary ordinance" (*testamentarisk förordnande*) (SOU 1984:79:281). This issue is not clearly regulated but it is an established praxis on a relatively limited scale (SOU 1984:79:281). Such an arrangement is different from legal personhood (legal agency) that may persist after death since the testament and wishes of the dead person are taken into consideration and are legally actionable. Thus, in accordance with the Autopsy Act, refusal of the patient prevails whenever it is not considered essential to establishing the cause of death, or if no criminal inquiry is called for.

Concepts and Principles Encoded in Laws

Individual Rationality and Consent

The (individual) person is understood as endowed with rationality and free-will, solely responsible for her actions.[215] Regarding the adult person's body the Swedish laws stress the person's full freedom to care for her health (and presumably her body) as she desires and to make decisions on the basis of her own judgement about measures to prevent or cure illness (Sjölenius 1989:59).

The person, defined as patient, in contact with Health Care institutions, is endowed with similar rights. The physician is supposed to be the patients' advisor and must accept the latter's decision. Legal justification is required in order to administer medical care without the individual's consent. However, the Health Care Act does not stipulate that consent to medical actions be mandatory. This is indirectly formulated in the demand that a patient has to be informed, treated with respect and that actions should be done in consultation with the patient.[216] The rationality of the patient cannot in principle be questioned, but the rationality of her action might be. Medical knowledge (and correct information) are important prerequisites to make a rational (and informed) decision. The degree of invasiveness or its consequences determine the importance in obtaining the consent of the patient.

The rational endowments of the person can be "temporarily" or more "permanently" lost. The conditions, of bodily (or mental) state in which the person is understood as temporarily mentally incapable, or only partially capable of rational judgements or behaviour, can concern states of unconsciousness or sedation, exhaustion etc. In these situations their consent to medical actions is presumed or regarded as tacit (if they did not previously express their disapproval). If the case is serious enough, the agency of the next-of-kin replaces (temporarily) the absent agency of the individual.

Even greater deprivation of agency is observable in the case of alcoholics or mentally ill. The result is a body without full personhood.[217] In these cases consent to medical actions is presumed or regarded as tacit if there are legal representatives available (Rynning, 1994:391). The (temporary) loss of rationality (and therefore agency) of the mentally ill calls for external agency. The relationship personhood-body is in part temporarily suspended. This holds also – but more permanently – for certain categories such as senile persons, very young children, and those defined as incompetent. These persons have less than full legal personhood, fewer legal rights and fewer mental responsibilities, "partial" actors. The bodies of these persons are dealt with as partial persons since they lack full capacity to understand how to act on behalf of their own interests. Thus, their bodies are protected by custodians or institutions. They are not allowed to make certain decisions (i.e. raising children), cannot sign contracts and cannot write testaments that are legally actionable. In short they are socially dis-abled.[218] Thus, the "will" of a person concerning her body may under certain circumstances be ignored by her family, medical professionals and other authorities.

In case that citizens (or residents) are defined as lacking proper mental competence or judgement capability – either temporarily or permanently – other agents are empowered to make the judgement on their behalf and to provide consent for medical actions (in some cases, this is done without legal basis, as pointed out above). In Sweden the next-of-kin seem to play a much more prominent role in giving consent than the law allows (Rynning, 1994). This is because medical personnel turn to them in situations where the patient's consent cannot be obtained, or when there is uncertainty about it (as in the case of necrodonation).

Physicians are the societal agents having the authority to judge if a person lacks personhood temporarily or permanently, for example to define them as mentally incompetent or ill – and also to define them as potentially dangerous to themselves and/or others. Such persons are thus subject to the determinations or decisions of others in giving consent to take medical actions on their bodies. Apparently, many medical interventions are taken without proper consent in the legal sense (Rynning, 1994). Such infringement can take place without any legal sanction, or with minimum disciplinary sanctions – presumably under the implicit assumption of "good intent and expertise". [219] Rynning (1994:399) points out:

> In practice, many health care procedures are based on such an artificial
> assumption about the patient's consent that they can hardly be regarded
> as compatible with demands of respect for patient's autonomy. It can
> also include situations of coercion without any support of laws or
> emergency. Commonly these measures take place in the care of

mentally disabled, senile demented and other patients with mental diseases.

Control rights over the person's body – rights distributed between the individual citizen and the state (hospitals and other authorities as agents) – largely favour the individual as long as the individual is alive and capable (but, as indicated, there are important exceptions, made for reasons of practical public good or health). But still the law sets certain limits on the person's full control over the body. While it allows an individual to "sell" certain parts (hair, blood) and to donate organs, there are restrictions on the individual's right to sell other parts or to determine how her donated organs are to be used or by whom. Sperm donors, for example, cannot determine recipients. Similarly, a person who decides to donate organs after her death may not determine recipients. Individuals are nevertheless allowed to determine which research institution receives her body for medical training.

Bodily Autonomy vs. Collective Interest

The *right to bodily integrity* is regarded as fundamental, and a key attribute of the person, who is entitled to exercise control over it. Consequently, she has the freedom to refuse authorities or persons to infringe on her body. Even if "protection of life" is an important value in the legislation, it does not take precedence over right to bodily autonomy. Under no circumstances can a mentally capable adult person be forced to receive medical care, even if it puts her life at risk. No medical actions can be exerted upon her without her consent. According to the Health Care Act, medical actions on patient's bodies must be carried out in consultation with the patient, informing the patient about the procedures and respecting her integrity and decisions. The Health Care Act has a general and indeterminate character concerning the rights and obligations of patients and health care personnel (Rynning, 1994:121). Still, medical actions on bodies of competent adult patients require consent. Oral consent in major procedures and silent consent for the simple or common procedures are the standard forms of consent (Rynning, 1994:322).

Besides Constitutional rights, the right to bodily autonomy has it strongest manifestation in the Abortion Act (1974:595). Any woman, independently of her age (but not independently of her level of rationality) is entitled to obtain an abortion without any restrictions, up to 12 weeks of pregnancy. No other agent (parent, custodian or husband) has the right to decide upon her body in this particular procedure. However, a physician can refuse to perform the operation if it threatens the woman life and health. A legally competent (rättskapabel) woman cannot be forced to follow any medical treatment to save the life and health of the foetus, even in a state of advanced pregnancy (Rynning, 1994:375).[220]

A woman is entitled to receive health care, and receive care in the form of insemination with donor sperm, and fertilisation outside the body, but consent of her husband is required (single women are not entitled to these procedures). In these particular procedures, in the name of the child's right to a good environment, the woman's rights are shared with the rights of the prospective child as well as with the (legal) father. Since the child is not yet born, the state acts as trustee. Such regulations are formulated on the basis of collective interests.

In case of important societal interests in carrying out a medical action upon somebody's body, severe limitations on the exercise of individual rights are applied. The safeguarding of societal values or the "common good" can be enacted through special regulations or in emergency.[221] The most common situation where integrity rights are suspended by reason of the common good is when a person suffers from mental disease (Act on Forced Confinement Under Psychiatric Care) or when a person carries a dangerous contagious disease (Act on Spreading of Infectious Diseases). In both cases a person can be held in a hospital and receive medical treatment against her will.[222] The LTP Act concerns the mentally ill, or persons with advanced degree of senility.[223] Examples of other situations where public good, risk, or safety are central and where exceptions to individual rights are made, concern violent or criminal persons, forensic controls, and cases of crime or suspected criminality in general, and protecting senile or mentally disturbed persons from harming themselves or disturbing others. In general, the more serious or important the public or collective interest in the medical action, the more likely that *individual rights are compromised or surrendered*.[224]

There is a tension between the organising idea or principle of individual (bodily) integrity and autonomy, and particular practical considerations and interests, for example the research interest of the medical profession or the health care interest of those administering hospitals and clinics. The existence of different principles (and interests) in the formulation of these laws explains some of the exceptions, compromises and inconsistencies about the treatment of the individual and her body. For example, the application of the Act for Prevention of Infectious Diseases to non-compliant HIV carriers or AIDS patients is an illustration of collective concerns in the suspension of bodily integrity.

The principle of citizen autonomy in the law also makes a concession to instrumental or practical goals which state agents have or support. Thus, the right of autonomy of adult citizens is circumscribed. Blood and small parts can be taken from bodies (including from living bodies in connection with operations). These are used for diagnosis and control (of operations), medical autopsies, forensic autopsies, transplantation, research. Clearly, the principle of bodily autonomy is not absolute. *Contradictory values underlie the laws as cultural products.* The resolution of such contradictions in the specific laws represents a particular social rationality. The purposes for which organ parts may be removed without the permission of the person are also formalised in the law. Some purposes are seen as more legitimate or central than others – that is with greater claim to compromise citizen's bodily autonomy: forensic autopsy or access to parts and tissue (e.g. blood) that are essential to the operation of modern medical systems.

All in all, however, rights to bodily integrity and autonomy of a person is an important principle in Swedish legislation. The person is equivalent to the adult individual, and she is assumed to be rational, to know what is good for her, to be capable of protecting her own interests and, accordingly, to be capable of making judgements. Thus, infringement on her body requires her consent – except if this interferes with the application of other important regulations and emergency. There is some coherence in the different rules and regulations relating to the citizen's body but this may not be through conscious design. They make up a highly complex, piecemeal construction of the body, reflecting various negotiations and compromises between different considerations and interests. The overall pattern is that, on the one hand, the general principle of the right of a citizen to personal and bodily integrity is present in a range of laws regulating medical and related treatment of bodies; on the other hand, *compromises and exceptions are made for purposes of common welfare* (e.g. exigencies of medical practices and research). Elsewhere (Machado, 1996b), I have referred to this pattern as *pragmatic principalism* (cf. Heclo, 1983), entailing a certain type of modern social rationality (Burns and Flam, 1987). One explanation for this rationality is that general universal principles tend to be applied directly or indirectly in each and every law bearing on citizens (and their bodies). There are also particular interpretations and negotiations in the formulation of each law. Here, particular interests, power configurations and arguments come into play and influence the outcomes of any given formulation process. In each case there are contextually specific influence processes, as well as more or less influential legal, technical, and moral discourses. These are not entirely pragmatic or opportunistic. Universal principles are applied insistently. But particularistic concerns (pragmatic, professional, partisan, etc.) enjoy some influence over specific formulations and applications without undermining or substantially compromising the universal principles. Out of this emerges not only a more or less common application of the universal principles, but some variation and inconsistency in the specific applications of the principle in legal formulations. Typically, such "reasoned" (or reasonable) inconsistency does not evoke major criticism or opposition, for there is a basic assumption of common good and also a "story of justification" for every exception or limitation that assumes a *basic rationality* (in Levi-Strauss' terms there is a myth around the processes of promulgation and amendment of Acts). The "stories" associated with, for example, the Transplant Act tell us that exceptions to the basic rationality are made because of "necessity", "emergency", or practicality – discourses such as "if blood were included in the Transplants Act the entire operation of a modern hospital would be jeopardised".

Conclusion: The Interaction of Law and Medicine

Legal institutions and discourses play a significant role in constructing disciplinary power relations and regulating action, in relation to such areas as work, family, the professions, education, and medicine. But Law is not singular or monolithic. It is complex, differentiated. It constrains, regulates, and disciplines. That is, there are coercive, if not repressive, aspects, but it also establishes legitimacy and guides action (Cohen and Arato, 1992). It provides openings and opportunities for autonomy, even for resistance, of the "rational" citizen. That is, it does not simply "inscribe" on the citizen's body *à la* Michel Foucault but provides opportunities for autonomy and resistance, in part in the zone of tension between individual autonomy and collective interest. In other words, modern civil and political rights are not simply ideology or deception but provide considerable protection of freedom and autonomy – even in relation to the disciplines and the exercise of "biopower". This relates to the explosion of civil rights consideration in our century (Cohen and Arato, 1992:263).

Hewitt (1991:229), drawing on some suggestions of Foucault, emphasises the linkages between the juridical system, and the disciplines and their technicians.[225] "However, rather than fade into the background, the law operates more and more as a norm, so that the judiciary is gradually incorporated into a continuum of apparatuses (medical, administrative, etc.) whose functions are regulatory." He refers to the notion of rights, which is central to modern democratic law: the rights to life, to one's body, to health, to happiness, to the satisfaction of needs.

My analysis stresses the Weberian idea of the centrality of rational conceptions of man and society in legal systems. The legislation process, especially in the area of technology, science, medicine, entails the mobilisation of experts in formulating laws, in preparing legislation that will enjoy legitimacy and function effectively (Turner, 1992). That is, the juridical area I examine here combines formal law with medicine. Cohen and Arato (1992:264) single out these "non-normative developments within law and legal discourses that are implicit in the modern structure of power". The use of medical, psychological, sociological expertise, of statistical data, in short of empirical information and non-legal languages within legal discourses to make one's case, is proof that the disciplines of science and empirical knowledge have penetrated the juridical structures and rendered them positive, functional, and quasi-disciplinary in character (Cohen and Arato, 1992:264). In the formulated laws, there are cultural assumptions, encodings about the rational citizen who has the capability to know what she wants, to choose, etc. In other words, citizens are constituted as "reasonable", "rational", "capable" beings in *particular terms*. This also means they are *knowable, calculable, and normal* – from the prospective of policy-makers, regulators, and the knowledge producers who serve them (Cohen and Arato, 1992: 268). Research on laws relating to medical actions on the body suggests a certain coherence and consistency to the laws, although there has been no systematic juridical effort at integrating all laws discussed in this chapter. There has been, however, recent attempts to integrate several of the laws (e.g. Transplantation, Dissection and Autopsy Acts dealing with medical actions on the body), but issues concerning the distinctions between living and necrodonation and current developments in reproductive technologies made these efforts problematic; and impeded the legal construction of a new unified Act.

10 Ethical Issues

Why Bioethics Today?

Ethical issues concerning the use of biotechnology are a major concern today, and consequently ethical guidelines are in high demand (Dubose et al., 1994; Fox, 1993; 1990, 1988; 1984; Toulmin, 1994). The current interest in ethics and normative guidelines is principally a result of the introduction of new medical (bio)technologies, that go beyond the reach of previously existing laws and norms, and for which new social regulations have to be instituted, concerning not only the proper use of such technologies but also the extent of public access and contribution to them. Other factors have also contributed to the increased role of ethics in medicine such as the mounting costs of health care systems that in most cases have brought about economic restrictions and managed care programs, but also rendered visibility to medical systems, and led to a closer examination of the procedures for rationing scarce medical resources. The visibility of medical decision-making has increased immensely in the context of growing rights of patients vis-à-vis medical procedures – or as consumers of health care services. Also, there is an intense media coverage of new developments in biotechnology as "human interest" stories. To this has to be added that "the physician" of today does not command the same professional [and moral] authority that (s)he had only some fifty years ago to decide alone about issues such as rationing of care, choice of treatment, or even the determination of death.

What can be morally or ethically problematic with organ transplantation?

(1) Organ transplantation evokes a whole complex of moral, professional, ethical and legal problems. In Chapter 6, I presented a model of the impact of a major technological development on clinical practice and law. The development not only crosses boundaries but generates new boundaries, ambiguities, predicaments, and issues relating to what is good or bad, right or wrong.

(2) It is morally and legally difficult to control a development where there is a powerful convergence of patient interest (in living, or at least radically improving the quality of life) and professional interest (in developing and applying new techniques and technologies, particularly ones

which are highly dramatic and even magical in character). And where this development often confronts and disturbs (or runs the risk of often confronting and disturbing) the deepest, often religious, sensibilities of human beings. As Moore (1988) clearly puts it:

> When capital gains, investor profit, institutional reputation, fame, surgeon ego, municipal pride and chauvinism become the objective of the procedure, then the ethical climate of the institution is no longer acceptable for therapeutic innovation.

(3) In law and medical formulations, one speaks of the "gift of life", but in a very practical sense, organ procurement programs are oriented to increasing "supply". But gaining access to and extracting organs runs the risk of violating the sensibilities of next-of-kin and the intentions of deceased persons. Typically, the question of "organ donation" must be discussed with disturbed next-of-kin. They are usually emotionally upset and preoccupied with dealing with the sense of loss. Of course, as in Spain, one may recruit and educate specialists who work with communicating with next-of-kin. But the Spanish type system runs the risk of *systematically* violating the sensibilities of next-of-kin (and the integrity of the deceased citizen).[226]

(4) Organ transplantation is a very expensive, high-technology treatment. One needs infrastructure, well-trained personnel, special laboratories, operation rooms, access to expensive medicines, and long follow-up regimes. When one compares organ transplantation to many cancer treatments, the method is effective and highly certain. On the other hand, should one allocate resources in such a way? In a global perspective, it is a technology for the rich countries and rich persons in the world.

Toward a Sociology of Ethics

Sociology stresses that what is considered "right" or "good" depends on the perspectives of the actors involved in the situations in which they act and interact. The term *actor* in this context points at another important sociological premise: people act in families, villages, cities, churches, communities, nations, and other groupings that are held together through human interaction, characterised by innovations, feelings, accidents and misunderstandings and fuzziness. There is another sociological premise important to point out: most people find themselves in – for them preexisting – social institutions. The institutions have not been intentionally created by them, but they shape and regulate their behaviour to a large extent. In a certain sense, institutions function as a set of premises for people (and as bases for other institutions) both as constraints and possibilities, providing the stuff for what they regard in many instances as obvious, natural, commonsensical and generally taken for granted. One finds, however, a tension between the quasi-natural character of many human institutions (a "naturalistic" orientation) and the movements and initiatives of human agents to reform or even transform such arrangements. In this tension lies the methodological and theoretical richness of much sociological analysis.

A sociological analysis focuses on the identification of the particular normative rules that apply to decisions and actions of the social agents (such as donors, professional staff, administrators, etc.) involved in a specific medical setting, for instance organ procurement. Social relationships and institutional domains are constituted and regulated by distinct, socially defined rule systems. Each rule system in an institutional domain involves not only specific organising principles and transaction rules, but a jurisdiction of meaning. It defines and distinguishes the legitimate actors (to be included, respectively excluded) in the collective activity, the type of actions and interactions to be performed in the setting, the appropriate or proper places and times to engage in the activity. Social rules systems constitute the grammars and semantics by which human beings relate to one another, deal with one another, and understand one another. From this perspective moral norms are understood as particular social rules.

1. In a hospital or clinical setting, some norms and values have a moral or sacred character. For example, there are principles concerning respect for the autonomy or integrity of a patient, or those relating to prioritisation of patients. Some of these may be formulated in laws or well-established policies. While they play a greater or lesser role in guiding decisions and actions, they are not the only determinants. Other factors in the situation enter in. Toulmin (1994:310) points out that in medical praxis (as in most other instances of decision-making) decision and action have technical as well as moral aspects. The technical side depends on *matters of judgement*, that is physicians' and nurses' experiences and perceptions of the situation. Such judgements are not usually verbalisable or reducible to "essential bare bones" to be ethically analysed in terms of abstract principles. Toulmin (1994:314) points out:

> The task of the medical casuist is, then, *to refer difficult cases arising in marginal or ambiguous situations to simpler, more nearly paradigmatic examples* and to consider how far the simpler examples can guide us in resolving the conflicts and ambiguities awakened. However, divisions among physicians regarding ethical issues typically arise because of *the details of the particular situation they confront*, e.g., cases of terminal illness either embodying conflicts between two or more coexisting

> demands about whose moral value all basically agree; or else arise at
> the margin of application of ideas (e.g. autonomy) about which there
> would have been no problem, *if the case in question had been
> paradigmatic – central and free of ambiguity.*

In the medical literature, there are many reports of particular discursive activities in hospital settings that address anguish, resolve contradictions and tensions, convey particular definitions and meanings of the situation.

2. The sociological perspective entails (1) socially embedding particular ethical principles, judgement processes and discourses in concrete interaction settings with particular institutional arrangements; (2) recognising that ethical considerations are but a part of a complex matrix of factors which enter into actors' decisions and practices. Both these considerations imply the necessity of conducting empirically oriented investigations of ethical processes: the actual ethical judgements, reflections, and decisions of agents in their medical contexts. The particular ethical rules and processes are socially embedded. One tries to identify the particular ethical principles or rules that actors consider relevant in the situation and are supposed to apply. These are not the only factors in their decisions and judgements. Sometimes actors cannot realise or implement their ethical rules; they lack the resources or there are constraints on them. Sometimes other values enter in and compel a compromise or negotiation. Thus one expects to find gaps or deviations between relevant ethical rules and actual judgements and practices.

Specific Ethical Issues in Organ Transplantation

Organ transplantation is largely assumed by many to be unconditionally "good", and that the more organs given, acquired, and transplanted the better the situation is, medically as well as morally (Fox, 1994:41). But, strangely enough, there are many ethical issues around brain death, organ procurement, recipient selection and transplantation in general. Organ replacement surgery requires for its legitimisation not only adequate technical knowledge and skill, but also a high ethical commitment because – given its particular design – it entails many risks, not only medical but also ethical ones. The following discussion drawing upon my own observations and investigations suggests several major ethical concerns and risks (of the probability of breaching an ethical principle or code) in connection with organ transplantation (Machado, 1996), and others (Fox, 1974, 1988, 1989, 1990, 1993; Michielsen, 1991; Simmons et al., 1977).

Important questions regarding the ethics of organ transplantation are:

1. To what extent is it morally acceptable to cause harm to a healthy person in order to help another, particularly in the case of minors and mentally disabled persons? To what extent can such a donation be free and informed, that is free of coercion?
2. To what extent do therapy ambiguities and the very uncertainties associated with brain death determination and organ procurement raise ethical issues?
3. To what extent ought the consent of the deceased be taken into account in the extraction of her organs after death? To what extent should the opinion of the kin count?
4. Is it ethically right to let a dying patient finally die in an operation theatre in order to extract organs immediately after death?
5. Is it right and proper to reimburse one way or another the relatives of a deceased donor? Is it permissible to allow a person to sell a kidney?
6. Who should be given priority in receiving an organ?
7. Should some categories of patients go before others on the waiting lists, such as children, adults supporting families, worthy citizens? Should alcoholics, drug addicts, prison inmates, mentally disabled or psychologically disturbed persons be accepted as organ receivers?
8. To what extent should one re-adjust or countervail "natural" imbalances or inequities occurring in blood and other types of matching? Or between men and women?

All these issues have in common being ethically and legally contested areas, and consequently have been discussed and analysed at length in various ethical discussion networks, publications and public forums.

Organ Procurement

According to the existing international guidelines concerning human organ transplantation – adhered to by most countries – organs for clinical transplantation are to be obtained through donation that is non-commercial procurement of organs and tissue. There are a number of ethical issues and problems connected with organ procurement. Some of these are recognised or intuited by lay persons. Popular perceptions of ethical risks associated with organ procurement often appear in the form of "metaphors of resistance", such as "the sinister organ bank" (in the film "Coma"), or widespread tales of "snatched kidneys" (such as stories of travellers that wake up the morning after a party to discover that one kidney is missing), and stories of children kidnapped for their organs or of corpses found in morgues without eyes, etc.

Living Organ Donation

Living organ transplantation includes the donation of kidneys, lobes of the lung, and segments of pancreas, liver, and the small intestine. The first successful solid organ transplantation in 1954 was made possible thanks to a kidney donated by the identical twin of the patient (genetically related living donors at that time proved the only viable way of avoiding organ rejection). The use of living donors is still widespread but raises ethical concerns inside and outside the medical profession. An official criticism of the utilisation of living organ donors was formulated by the Council of Europe (1967), recommending   that this type of donation should be restricted and if possible eliminated. Common arguments raised by medical professionals and ethicists who approve the utilisation of living donors are: the shortage of cadaver kidneys, the low risk for the health of the donor, and the excellent transplantation results obtained (Bos and Wilmink, 1991) (C. Bergström, 4/1996). Among the widely recognised ethical concerns related to living organ donation, four will be discussed here.

Primum Nihil Nocere: An important medical principle is not to inflict harm on a patient (for example through a surgical operation). The removal of an organ does not bring any benefit to the health of an organ donor but rather a physical injury. However, it is considered more or less acceptable to harm the donor as long as the injury is limited, and the purpose is to alleviate or save the life of a next-of-kin. Where the line goes between ethical or unethical harming is principally defined by the laws of the respective countries where this is applied. For example, while the Swedish legislation puts the limit at "serious risks" to the donor, the Danish legislation goes further and puts the limit where *"direct danger* to the donor arises"(Akveld and de Charro, 1991:45). The ethical and legal rule of not inflicting serious risk to, or at least avoiding a serious endangerment of, the donor's health is clear, *but application of the rule is a matter of medical interpretation, and medical opinions are divided.* Even if the mortality figure for living donors is fairly low, the surgical and long term risks for organ donors, particularly kidney donors, are not negligible (Michielsen, 1991).

The medical justification for inflicting an injury on a healthy living donor is the advantage of good tissue compatibility in living donation. However, the superiority of organ donation between blood relatives (e.g. parents and children) when compared with similar cadaver tissue matching has been questioned by McMaster & Czerniak (1991). Good transplantation results are also achievable through a systematic selection of the recipients of necroorgans.[227] The increased use of non-genetically related living donors (see Bos and Wilmink,1991) indicates that it is not so much medical but social policy oriented criteria which are often utilised in approving living organ donation.

In sum, the ethical balance "high benefit to the organ recipient and minor injury to the organ donor" depends on a non-ethical technical judgement: the estimated success of an organ transplantation, and the estimated low risk to the donors. Since such assessments depend on a number of systemic factors extended over a period of time, the acceptable ratio benefit/injury cannot be readily calculated, making the determination of ethical balance or trade-off difficult if not impossible.

The risks of breach of informed consent: Modern transplantation laws emphasise the voluntary and informed character of donation. Sells (1991) attributes the character of Western legislation to the principles stated in the codes of Nuremberg (1974) and Helsinki (1964) stressing the principles of free choice and informed consent in medical procedures. Thus, the rule of *informed consent* is included in most legislation.[228] The principle of informed consent involves ethical values such as individual autonomy and self-determination. Adequate information, regarded as a prerequisite of the consent, requires sufficient cognitive sophistication to enable the individual to properly judge the balance of the procedure's benefits and damages. However, the application of this rule is subject to several practical considerations. There are reasons to doubt the ideal application of the doctrine of presumed consent:[229] it is assumed that the organ donor understands the short and long term effects of the procedure. This assumption have been challenged by several empirical studies, particularly in the case of lay donors without technical knowledge, or persons having a substantially different social and cultural background from the physician.[230] Living organ donation in most OECD countries is safeguarded by strict legal demands of consent (e.g. written consent) favouring a more rigorous praxis than for the normal patient. Still, precisely how this is implemented in transplantation centres is an empirical question. Another important point is the lack of general consensus among physicians about the risks involved in live organ donation (Michielsen,1991). This implies that the particular opinion or judgement of the responsible physician will affect the information that the potential donor receives and utilises in order to reach an "informed" decision regarding organ donation. In sum, the social conditions surrounding judgement and decision-making in living organ donation contribute to a greater or lesser extent to ethical risks.

The issue of children and mentally handicapped acting as organ donors is particularly controversial because the principles of voluntary and informed consent are obviously not met. Since medical considerations (e.g. tissues compatibility) can justify the use of these donors, the practice is allowed but mainly for renewable tissue (e.g. bone marrow). The restriction on the use of children-donors is intended to protect them from abuse. But there are also restrictions on donations from older children, whose opinion for many medical procedures, at least in Sweden, is otherwise taken into consideration around puberty (Rynning, 1994).

The risk of pressures to donate: Studies of living organ donation show that living organ donation more than altruistic giving is a form of "gift exchange" (Simmons et al., 1977) according to rules of giving and reciprocity established in the family. These studies suggest that living organ transfers are less the expression of a free decision to donate than a result of sentiments, obligations and familial negotiations. Family pressures to donate are not uncommon, and it is difficult for a transplantation surgeon to assess whether or not a particular organ donation is the result of such pressures (Bergström, 1994). All these factors indicate the contextual and negotiated character of much organ donation, and the importance of attending to the institutional and cultural context in which the decisions take place.

Commercialised donation: Commercialisation of living organ donation is regarded as deeply unethical in OECD and most other countries, and commodification of organs is regarded as a real risk in such transfers. Not surprisingly, commercial transactions with organs for transplantation are legally banished in OECD and many other countries. The rules applied in this matter are ethical, on the one hand, and pragmatic, on the other. The ethical principles refer to justice, individual autonomy, human dignity and avoidance of human commodification. Common normative criteria applied are illustrated in a quotation from Abuna et al., 1991:

> *[The commercialisation of organ donation has]*...a negative impact on public voluntarism and altruism, increases the risk of exploitation of the poor (by private hospitals, physicians), deprecates fundamental professional and moral values of society by demeaning the dignity and the autonomy of the human individual... It promotes an unjust system of organ access and distribution controlled by market forces which favours the rich.

Some pragmatic approaches condone human tissue markets (cf. organs) if there are no risks of low quality.[231] But donation motivated by altruism is a means of assuring quality control, as argued by Titmuss (1970) in the case of blood donation (see discussion in Chapter 3).

However, it is not difficult to draw a clear line between commercialisation and "rewarded gifting". Accepted monetary reimbursement for temporary loss of working capacity and travelling costs are not uncommon in some countries. A practical consideration is the difficulty, especially for a transplantation surgeon, to assess that the terms of organ donation exclude monetary exchange or other gains. In general, there are serious risks and a very slippery slope.

Necrodonation

In necrodonation important ethical concerns arise in connection with establishing rules regulating such donations and dealing with the various risks of violating human sensibilities.[232] [233]

The forms of donation: In the OECD countries, the most common form of organ procurement is through necrodonation. The terms of the donation are often written in the transplantation laws of the respective countries, or at least established through national medical guidelines. The rules for cadaveric organ donation range between presumed consent and non-presumed consent, with more or less strict interpretations of these principles; no OCED legislation prescribes the compulsory extraction of cadaver organs. The principle of *presumed consent* for cadaveric organ donation states that organs and tissue can be extracted from a deceased, as long as the deceased while alive, had not expressed [either in written or verbal form] a refusal to donate. The rule of *non-presumed consent* for cadaveric organ donation states that organs and tissue can be extracted from a deceased, as long as the deceased while alive, had expressed a positive attitude to organ donation either in written or verbal form (see Chapter 3). There are important ethical and practical differences between these principles:

(a) Presumed consent emphasises notions of social solidarity, and is based on the notion that to donate organs *is* the norm, and consequently a refusal to donate is a *negative deviation* from the norm.[234] Since this norm is viewed as a positive act, the deviation becomes a negative and egoistic act. Instead of altruism, one articulates a notion of a quasi-civic duty in donating organs, grounded on notions of social solidarity in society. Ethically, presumed consent rules increase the risk of extracting body parts from people who do not want to donate, transforming presumed consent into organ expropriation and potentially de-legitimising the whole procedure.[235] For this reason, presumed consent legislation typically allows, for those individuals who do not want to donate, to inscribe their attitude in a register, or simply to express their wishes to relatives. Registers and family attestations are supposed to be safeguards against the risk of organ expropriation. It is assumed that those individuals who refuse to donate will be motivated enough to let their opinions be known. Of course, this does not need to be the case. Undecided individuals, or those slightly negative towards donation, can choose to postpone the decision until they make up their minds about the matter. Also, not everyone makes family manifestos about cadaveric organ donation or carries a donor card. The ethical balance in presumed consent entails querying to what extent the principle of helping patients in need of transplantation justifies steps that lead to other ethical risks. The argument that organ donation saves lives and alleviates suffering is too powerful an argument. It stops discussion and is not apt to evoke any public policy discussion other than that of an utilitarian variety. Most OECD countries have presumed consent policies. In spite of the explicit goal of presumed consent policy to increase the supply of organs, the Partnership for Organ Donation (a Boston-based non-profit organisation) found that the number of donors per million population is fairly similar among OECD including USA. They conclude that educating health professionals to recognise potential donors and to initiate the donation process as well as skilful communications that respond to the needs of families are the key to increasing organ donations (Newsletter, 1994).[236]

(b) Non-presumed consent emphasises notions of individual autonomy and integrity and is based on the notion that to donate organs *is not* the general norm.[237] Consequently, cadaveric donation *is a positive deviation from the standard norm*, thus becoming an altruistic action. The same action – donating organs – that in the case above has neutral value, acquires here a positive value, solely as a result of shifting the context normality. The risk involved in this form of consent concerns the issue of letting patients die on waiting lists because the number of people prepared to donate is low. However, according to the Partnership for Organ Donation, this argument does not hold (see paragraph above).

Commercialisation: Is it permissible to reimburse the relatives of a deceased donor? The possibility of promoting organ donation with the help of financial incentives has been discussed. Expressed ethical concerns are the potentially decreased emotional gain for the donor family, and the risk of a decreased respect for life and the sanctity of the human body. Great concern has also been expressed regarding a potential rich-versus-poor phenomena and the fact that financial need should not be linked in a coercive way to giving consent for organ procurement (Nelson et al., 1993).

Brain Death

The adoption of brain death criteria in establishing death improved the transplantation of kidneys and made possible transplantations of heart, livers, lungs, etc. However, the determination of death as the total and irreversible loss of all cerebral functions has been subject to controversies inside and outside the medical profession (Horton and Horton, 1991:1048; De Vita and Snyder, 1993:136; De Vita, Snyder and Gränvik, 1993; 113-129; Veatch, 1993; Brante and Hallberg, 1989). Death is certified after establishing that brain functions are absent and that this state is practically irreversible.[238] Several ethical issues have been raised regarding this concept of death.

Expanded death: According to the initial postulates that gave support to the "Harvard Criteria", brain death is an unstable clinical condition that leads to circulatory collapse within a few hours or days at the most. However, in several cases – not all that surprising considering today's sophisticated technology – cardiocirculatory functions have been maintained more than six months after the certification of cerebral death, and apparently well over one year in infants. This calls into question the extent to which the accepted criteria of brain death meets a culturally acceptable notion of death.

Legal-medical discrepancy in the determination of death: Standard medical tests do not guarantee that *all* brain functions have actually ceased. Legal requirements are thus not always met in clinical practice, creating many times a situation of ethical anxiety in the medical and nursing personnel and a legal-medical discrepancy.

Irreversibility: One of the main criteria in brain death diagnosis is the criterion of irreversibility. However, it appears that it is not possible to determine the exact point at which auto-resuscitation (i.e. *reversibility*) will not occur in humans (De Vita et al., 1993). The latter (De Vita et al., 1993:382) states:

> Reversibility... is a moral concern only if the patient and/or the physician chooses resuscitation. Although technically possible, resuscitation is in practice not available to the patient because of prior decisions, thus the possibility of resuscitation is morally irrelevant, and the patient is irreversible dead when auto-resuscitation will not occur.

In other words "irreversibility" may be contingent on human choice, for example the choice of withholding measures which might have proven effective.

Diagnostic accuracy?: Errors in determining brain death are unlikely, in principle. However, the skill of physicians in determining death may vary, particularly if the hospital has little experience with brain death cases. Apparently EEG measurements are not extremely reliable in meeting criteria of brain death (Veatch, 1993a), and measurement of the blood circulation in the brain may not be mandatory and is applied only in certain cases (for example, in Sweden).

Ethical/cognitive ambiguity: (a) The measures needed for the preparation of a potential donor, prior to the determination of death (e.g. heparinisation, draping of the patient) are not meant to benefit the patient. Moreover, the preventive measures required for an optimal maintenance of vital organs other than the brain, can be – at least in principle – counterproductive to an eventual recovery of a potential donor; (b) It may be difficult for ICU personnel to generally accept the fact that they are carrying out extreme measures to preserve an organ, not sustain a person alive (see Chapters 6 and 7). Since benefit to the braindead is absent, a certain ethical ambiguity may be experienced in maintaining the donor's organs in good condition (a fairly technically demanding procedure). In sum, high-tech death entails a number of ethical issues and risks which have yet to be fully and satisfactorily addressed.

Prioritisation and Selection of Patients

Should some categories of patients go before others in receiving organs. And, if so, what criteria should be used in determining such allocation. Given the substantial shortage of organs, *allocation rules make a difference. In principle, they should elicit a sense of fair selection*, given the public character of organ allocation systems. A stress on values associated with objective standards of allocation, and non-discrimination in allocation with respect to age, sex, gender, race and religion is fundamental. However, there are multiple competing principles of fair and proper allocation, as pointed out in Chapter 4. If we examine, for instance, the explicit criteria of UNOS or Eurotransplant, they appear to try to find some balance between *HLA matching* (stressing the immunological advantages of tissue compatibility) and *waiting time* (stressing the efficiency of modern immunosuppression and fairness to infrequently matched patient groups). The balance shifts over time. Analytically, this can be seen as an a compromise between medical utility and equity. Other problems and issues regarding selection are the following:

(1) *Selection as a process depending on multiple actors and multiple judgements.* Judgements concerning the allocation of organs are typically complex and difficult. (a) The selection of patients does not take place solely at the transplantation centre but also at local levels. The selection indirectly depends on factors such as the stage of the disease at which a patient is admitted to a the waiting list (patients with less health deterioration have a better chance of recovery). Since patients are commonly admitted to a list by recommendation of the local physician (following a pre-transplantation assessment), his/her opinion will affect when and if a patient is registered. Even highly centralised systems entail a number of local judgements, e.g. the urgency of a patient's state or the judgements leading up to (or not leading up to) placement on a waiting list – many potential recipients never make it to the transplantation centre. Thus, decisions about allocation take place well before a potential recipient becomes the concern of a particular transplantation program. (b) The process of selection at the transplantation centre comprises both admission to the waiting list and subsequent ranking of candidates. The admission and ranking of patients in transplantation lists varies from centre to centre. It is primarily based on biomedical criteria (e.g. urgency, compatibility between organ and receiver) and secondarily on psychosocial (e.g. the non-compliant patient) and fairness and administrative criteria (e.g. first come first served). Even if biomedical criteria are regarded as the most neutral ones, they are not devoid of ethical implications. For instance, the emphasis on antigen matching in ranking transplantation candidates contributes to increased waiting times (and mortality) for people with rare antigens (e.g. Black Americans in the US). It is a matter of the extent to which one is justified in risking a less than perfect matching if it is outweighed by some physical deterioration of the patients waiting on the list.

(c) The process of allocation of organs comprises at least two dimensions, the proper selection of patients and the organ allocation. While the "selection proper" means distributing an organ between several individuals, the allocation process also concerns distributing an organs/services between several institutions (i.e. giving equal access to organs to all hospitals of the region served by a transplantation centre). In these cases, a fair distribution of organs means to take into account both the individual and institutional levels.

(2) *Behavioural factors considered in the selection of patient.* Social, psychological, and other behavioural factors are taken into account, at least informally, in selection procedures, particularly in the selection prior to placement on waiting lists. It is generally recognised that such factors contribute to transplantation success. However, there is a general

ambivalence and reluctance among physicians involved in transplantation to utilise criteria that are diffuse and not strictly legitimised by medicine. Lack of confidence and competence to apply such criteria plays a role here. For example, one physician when interviewed explained: "These are very tricky things, and it's not a great idea to establish definite limits on paper about who is going to receive what". The medical profession tend to take their medical criteria as value-free, objective tools. On the other hand, they tend to feel that considerations of social and psychological factors are value- laden and threaten to undermine professional consensus.

Risk patients are understood as risky in a particular socio-cultural context. The abuse of substances (e.g. alcohol) is connected to what is considered socially to be acceptable levels of consumption. The male risk patient, who risks a longer period of rehabilitation because of the deprivation implied in a long disruption of his working activities, cannot be understood outside the frame of a social situation where the working role is still a major factor in constructing male identity. The same can be said for the perception of females as more successful recipients in that they tend to follow long term medicine regimes better than males do. The teenager recipient is perceived as a risk related to bodily changes. The prioritisation criteria also reflect to the explicit goal of the health system to totally rehabilitate the patient and integrate her socially into a normal life.

(3) *Local versus global access to organs.* A common problem in all organised systems is a tension between a centre and local or peripheral units concerning the control of resources and policy determinations. This includes the issue of distributive justice (in the allocation of organs) between a global unit and local units. Some systems recognise this as a problem from the outset and institutionalise a type of "sharing principle" as in Eurotransplant or in France Transplant. In addition, Scandiatransplant as well as UNOS have institutionalised "payback" principles. The various reciprocity or payback rules relate to systematic or global exchange rather than interpersonal. These are viewed as essential in establishing or maintaining a type of organisational distributive justice or fairness. In Eurotransplant, one takes into account in the point system the import/export balance. In the United States and in Scandiatransplant, there are rules specifying payback of organs within a certain time period.

(4) *Natural inequality and social rules of re-equilibration.* As pointed out in Chapter 4, "natural inequalities" arise because of the incompatibilities and unequal frequencies of blood groups. For instance,

persons with type O blood are universal donors, but may receive only from O donors. A not uncommon practice is to compensate for these inequalities through rules and regulations of selective allocation. Thus, because type O potential recipients tend to accumulate, waiting for a suitable donor, some allocation systems prescribe that type O organs should go first to type O recipients.

(5) *Gender and selection.* Many people are particularly sensitive to any inequities arising in connection with gender (or also class, ethnicity, race, region). As indicated in Chapter 3, females are significantly greater living donors than males. For instance, in Norway in the period 1988-92, females were 60% of the donors while males were 40%. On the other hand, women (as well as girls) were only 44% of the recipients. In general, males make up a higher proportion of recipients of cadaveric organs, although in this case they are significantly greater necrodonors than females (see Chapter 3). Official medical policies and pronouncements state that potential recipients of both sexes, are treated equally – although there are apparent imbalances. Some even suggest that in the organ allocation women are discriminated against (concerning hearts see Self and Olivarez, 1993). On the other hand, as I have shown, the selection of recipients and the allocation of organs are complex processes with many factors that affect the processes and their outcomes. Thus, the observable pattern that women are less likely than men to undergo, for instance, heart transplant may not necessarily be because of a gender bias in the selection processes, but because women are less likely to join such programs or are more disposed than men to refuse the surgery. In one study of 295 men and 91 women under the age of 70 who were candidates for heart transplantation, almost 30 percent of the women refused to go through with the operation compared to 9 percent of the men. While the question of gender inequity is a major public issue – making it very actual for organ allocation – any assessment of the type and degree of inequity must await a systematic study of how gender enters into and plays a part in the complex mechanisms of selection (as well as donation).

(6) *Levels of justice and scarcity.* The scarcity of organs available for transplantation is one of the most important constraints on allocation and the realisation of one or more principles of justice. Few causes of death fit the requirements for organ harvesting (that is, death caused by cerebral damage that leaves intact and "healthy" organs for transplantation). The greater the gap between supply and demand for organs, the more the pressure on decision makers to establish or redefine the criteria used in selection of recipients for organ transplantation, for example increasing stringency of selection.[239] This is a coping strategy which focuses

attention on risky patients, or patients that do not score high on all relevant criteria.

Whenever the demand for organs far exceeds the supply, one chooses "top patients", making selection criteria more stringent. This also would be expected to improve transplantation results. The selection of good patients for transplantation is regarded as one of the main factors in transplantation success. The generous criteria in selection of recipients applied in Sweden (for example patients up to 75 years may receive a graft organ) is explained by the short waiting lists. Even if the waiting time, e.g. for kidney transplantation, has extended from 6 months to two years still there is a relative lack of pressure due to low imbalance of supply and demand.

When the number of candidates for transplantation increases, as a result of less stringent selection criteria, the waiting time increases if the number of available organs remains constant or declines. This eventually poses the problem of how to regulate the dynamics of this system, avoiding inefficiently long queues and large numbers of untreated patients, or a system that will absorb more and more health care resources.

Ethics in a Systemic Perspective

A sociological analysis of the ethical dilemmas encountered in connection with organ transplantation – in contrast to philosophical normative analysis – focuses on the identification of the particular normative rules that apply to decisions of the social agents in different institutional domains.[240] In this perspective moral norms are understood as particular social rules. Social rules constitute the grammars by which social action and interaction are structured *but some of these social rules acquire the status of strong moral principles with "sacred", emotional connotations and deep commitments to them.* The particular institutional domains – with specific principles and priorities – exhibit also a particular bounded rationality and implicitly or explicitly a corresponding *bounded morality.*

An important factor in understanding the many ethical dilemmas encountered in the OTS is the social, organisational and normative complexity that characterises it. This is not only the result of the combination of medical and infrastructural technologies, but also the result of the heterogeneity of *actors* involved at different levels (physicians and other professional groups, relatives of deceased potential donors as well as groups of potential recipients, transplantation centres, sets of hospitals within harvesting areas, national and international organ exchange agencies, administrators, and so forth); and the *heterogeneity of social relationships* (administrative, professional, market, network-exchange, etc.) combined in the OTS.[241] For example, in an OTS the administrative concerns and responsibilities of a hospital administration differ from the concerns and duties professed by the different professional networks (see Chapter 5). They also differ from the concerns and duties of the families of organ donors, and also from the concerns and duties of the organ recipient with the new organ or "gift of life". On the one hand, the boundaries of the various institutional domains do not have to be closed or well defined (moreover, social domains have some values and norms in common, or apparently similar all-embracing goals). On the other hand, actors have the possibility of modifying and re-interpreting those moral rules.

Complexity, Heterogeneity and Ethical Systems

Max Weber in his sociology of ethics (Weber, 1977) identifies and discusses two different and irreconcilable types of ethical systems, the ethics of ultimate ends or "ethics of conviction", and the "ethics of responsibility". The ethics of conviction are unambiguous and uncompromising. The commitment to moral values and principles takes precedence over considerations of the outcomes of action, or over purely pragmatic considerations. It is the morally right action that is central, not particular outcomes – the latter in the end are disregarded. In contrast – and fitting to complex, modern societies and organisations – the ethics of responsibility takes real conditions into account, and thus includes instrumental considerations of efficiency and the means to be utilised. Ethical conflict is recognised and dealt with as a challenge (trying to find the least harmful solution). Weber points out that *the ethics of conviction (a type of fundamentalism) is particularly incompatible with modernity since it disregards the consequences or outcomes of the action, discounting effectivity and questions of efficiency.* The ethics of responsibility is particularly adapted to modern conditions, because it clearly recognises complexity and plurality of moral worlds.

Weber's conception of an ethics for modernity fits many of the conditions of OTS, where actors may not adhere *strictly* to a given moral rule. Typically, this has to do with other values or situational conditions, which the responsible or participating actors feel must be taken into account. For example, take the case of a potential necro-donor, who expressed a willingness to donate before death, but whose next-of-kin oppose this, and where the physician honours the sentiments of the family and does not proceed with organ removal, thus violating the will of the deceased. Or a transplantation clinic that decides not to take the first patient according to the waiting list, but to take a patient lower down on the list because the patient comes from a hospital which has contributed many organ donors and has not received as many organ transplants in return. Or a physician who determines that, although she should do everything possible for her patient, cannot prioritise her patient because it would mean going ahead of other patients in greater need or with greater probability of successful recovery.

Each example of deviation from a particular normative principle (and adherence to other principles) in actual practices, is common, and in many instances is justified or legitimised through particular discourses and understandings (see Chapter 8). But some deviations entail ethical risks, which may involve breaches that are eventually recognised and sanctioned. Some justifications, for example, in allocation of heart, kidney or liver to a patient from a hospital who is not high on the waiting list, because that hospital, more than other hospitals in the region, has been conscientious about providing organs but has received much less in return, cannot be maintained or defended publicly. But, obviously, the norm of reciprocity in a hospital exchange network is important for effective operating relationships and corresponds to a principle of distributive justice on the institutional level.

Many examples can be drawn from the clinical setting, where particular norms and values – some having a moral or sacred character – are applied to a concrete case or situation at hand. For example, there are principles concerning respect for the autonomy or integrity of a patient, or those relating to prioritisation of patients. Some of these may be formulated in laws or well-established policies and, while they play a greater or lesser role in guiding decisions and actions, *they are not the sole determinants of an action*. Given the complexity of circumstances and values to be taken into account, many factors enter into judgements and actions. This is not surprising since in *medical praxis* (as in most other areas of decision-making) *both decision and action have technical as well as moral aspects*. The technical side depends to a great extent on physicians' and nurses' expertise and professional judgement of the situation. Such judgements are not always verbalisable or reducible to "essential bare bones" to be ethically analysed in terms of a few abstract principles.[242]

Ethics of Responsibility as Pragmatic Principalism

The ethics of responsibility and pragmatic principalism (Machado, 1996b) are characterised by a strong commitment to ethical principles, but also by consideration of the complexity of the environment, of scientific "facts", of practical problems and issues, etc. Also, various legitimate interests have the right to make demands and to participate in the interpretations and deliberations, negotiations. In many legislative discussions and responses to biotechnical demands, e.g. organ transplantation,[243] the principle of individual rights over the body and its parts come under challenge (since human substance is extremely valuable for research and therapy). Examples of this type of problematic ethic are found in the Swedish legislation. Until 1996, minor organs and tissues could be extracted from a deceased during autopsy, without prior consent of the deceased or the relatives. This had to do with consideration of the *practical problems* that requesting consent would create (SOU, 1989:98). Also the recent legislation of presumed consent responds to concerns other than the principle of individual self-determination of the citizen, that is, the collective need for organs for transplantation, cost reduction and the harmonisation of the Swedish organ transplantation system with other European systems.

However, this pattern should not be confused with ad hoc or opportunistic or purely pragmatic considerations. These would make for ethically unacceptable policies as well as discourses. The intention is to formulate laws as well as policies that work, that will be effective regulators that will embody key principles. While a pure ethics of conviction would appear to provide an unacceptable basis of judgement, at least for medical and other scientific judgements and action, some degree of such ethics would seem necessary in complex modern societies. Above all, one must sustain core sacred values essential to the social order. Sacrality concerns a relationship between human actors and those principles, symbols, rituals, objects, and persons, that they define as sacred, deserving of reverence, non-negotiable, in a certain sense absolute (as opposed to the profane which is openly subject to calculation and instrumental considerations, negotiation and in general irreverence (Burns,1994:164)). Such a core of sacrality gives a community its identity, its vitality, perhaps its "spirit" or "soul".

Conclusion

To a certain extent modern medical science and practice tends to push and shove against moral boundaries, generating deep concerns inside and outside the medical profession. But moral or ethical concerns take place in circumstances where other norms also weigh heavily (e.g. increasingly effective ways of treating disease). Also criteria other than medical or ethical norms imbue the settings where judgement and decision-making take place. Consequences do not necessary reflect the intentions or the wishes of the actors themselves; they can be the unintended results of existing hospital routines, circumstances regarding the different technical demands for the type of organ to be implanted, accessibility to those organs/tissue and adequate technical and material resources, etc.

However, and for what concerns the large-scale systems of organ transplantation – even if compromises with efficiency is the predicament of a modern "responsible" ethics – it is important to remember Renée Fox's remark that "damage to the humane and moral foundations of the entire society can result from placing greater value on meeting the needs of organ recipients than on protecting donors, respecting the rights of persons, and protecting the vulnerable". And that perhaps it is not only the shortage of organs donated but the also the excess of transplants performed that has given rise to urgent concerns about "supply", "demand", and "organ shortfall". Again, there are several moral and ethical risks in the development of organ transplantation or in any large-scale technological development that penetrate many areas of our personal and social lives.

In sum, a sociological perspective on bioethics entails (1) socially embedding particular ethical principles, judgement processes and discourses in concrete interaction settings with particular institutional arrangements as well as shared cognitive-normative frames; (2) recognising that ethical considerations are but a part of a complex matrix of factors which enter into actors' judgements and practices. Both these considerations imply the need for empirically oriented investigations of ethical processes – the actual ethical reflections, judgements, and decisions of agents in any given institutional context. Since ethical rules and processes are socially embedded, one tries to identify the particular ethical principles or rules relevant or applying in the situation. While the participating actors apply the ethical rules – and refer to them in many of their discourses – these are not the only factors in their decisions and judgements. Sometimes, actors cannot realise or implement ethical principles; they lack the resources or there are constraints on them. Sometimes other values enter in and there is a process of situational compromise or negotiation. In general, a sociological approach to ethical processes prepares us to recognise and explain possible gaps or deviations betwen relevant ethical rules and actual ethical jugements and practices.

Appendix: Data Sources

Given the character of my research, a variety of methods have been employed in the collection of data: interviews, observations, studies of legal documents, surveys of newspapers and medical journals, selection and compilation of national and international statistical data, and investigation of relevant literature concerning not only the extensive and specialised material on organ transplantation but also on the process of medicalisation of society, instrumental rationality in modernisation processes, disciplination of bodies and related studies of cultural and technical change.

The data based on semi-structured interviews and observations was collected during the period 1990-1995 within the framework of a research project, directed by Tom R. Burns. Besides myself, Tom. R. Burns, Mats Hansson, Thorsten Rehn, Caroline Sutton and Johan Åhlfeldt were involved in collecting data, conducting interviews and making observations. The observations were carried out in the period 1991 to 1994 by myself and Johan Ahlfeldt. During this same period, 30 interviews (of 1-2 hours each) were conducted in Sweden with a wide variety of key actors: chiefs of transplantation clinics, transplant surgeons, anaesthesiologists, nurses, and assistant nurses. In addition to individual interviews, four group interviews with anaesthesiologists from intensive care units and with experience in organ retrieval were conducted by Burns, Hansson and Åhlfeldt.

Outside of Sweden, I conducted interviews with officials at Eurotransplant (Leiden, Holland) and Scandiatransplant (Arhus, Denmark) as well as OPO of the Washington, DC hospital consortium, USA. The interviews carried out in the USA included the head physician of a large intensive care unit, an ethicist, a lawyer specialised in transplantation policies, a transplantation co-ordinator and organ co-ordinators of the Organ Procurement Agency of the Washington hospital consortium. I also participated as an observer in a meeting between physicians of an intensive care unit and one of the ethicists of a Washington hospital. These interviews and observations gave me the possibility to gain a broader perspective on and insight into Swedish transplantation arrangements.

Besides data from observations, interviews and material presented in the sociological, medical and ethical literature, another important source of data – regarding the importance and generality of some of the problems analysed in the studies – was a discussion forum in the Internet (Mcw-Bioethics) originating at Yale University (USA). The forum consisted mainly of ethicists, physicians and lawyers and concerned issues of medical ethics. It provided a context where I could discuss and test out a number of my ideas and working hypotheses. I also participated in another Internet discussion forum (Trnsplnt) formed by patients either already transplanted or waiting for transplants, together with medical personnel and officials involved in transplantation activities.

In general, a hospital is a hierarchical, male-dominated organisation. Although a majority of the employees are women, men are typically in charge of the organisation. These features were no less pronounced in the surgical wards with which I had contact. This certainly affected how I was perceived and, on occasion, treated. For instance, once I was introduced – very affably – by a surgeon to an administrator of the hospital as "a girl (*flicka*) who will ask some questions". Another time I experienced hospital patriarchy in less affable circumstances. A leading transplantation surgeon stopped an interview I was conducting with a transplantation co-ordinator nurse because he felt that, as the nurse's superordinate, he should have been previously contacted by my project leader. He demanded that, before any further interviewing be conducted, the project leader would make contact with him. He also lectured me at length about his concept of science and the importance of statistical measurement in scientific research while questioning the scientific value of semi-structured interviews, such as the one I was conducting. Over time, I developed strategies to deal with such attitudes.

A reflection on my observations and interviews was the general and often intense concern with ethical issues among transplantation physicians and anaesthesiologists. Concurrently, there was a marked sensitivity to the possible "damages" that unfavourable information about organ transplantation could generate and the harm that this could cause in public opinion. These understandable medical concerns called for a sometimes tense and cautious research attitude on my part, since I was repeatedly made aware of my responsibility in the questions I asked and the formulations I made. It was stressed that I could otherwise bring harm to the patients and undermine public trust in the medical organisation.

Notes

1. A decontextualisation such as this is exemplified by the peculiar concept of the biomort. A biomort is a braindead, whose body is kept alive by means of life support systems, and it has been used to test drugs, uterine functions, and mechanical hearts (Moore, 1988). Its potential is estimated as large because it physiologically resembles an anaesthetised patient, and it can be used by medical students to learn surgical procedures, by researchers to test drugs and equipment. It is a stable, "no-risk organism" (Moore, 1988).

2. A later book Spare Parts (Fox and Sweazy, 1989) continues the examination of several of the issues taken up in The Courage to Fail, confirming that issues they had approached twenty years earlier were still of major significance: the endemic problem of how to allocate scarce resources, the shortage of organs due to the increased size and scope of transplantation, the importance of giving, and the medical and cultural furore by which organ transplantation has been driven and developed. An overall characteristic of the writings of Fox as well as Simmons and their associates is that a particular set of sociological concepts has played a major role in the analyses of not only organ transplantation but other bio-medical and related bioethical subjects. Key concepts that they have used – in addition to values, norms, statuses, roles, institutions, socialisation, and the like that are the building blocks of any sociological analysis – are uncertainty, ambiguity, detached concern, gift and gift exchange, the experiment-therapy dilemma, and structures and processes of social control (Fox, 1988:442). An important piece of sociological work is Simmons, Klein and Simmons' book The Gift of Life (Simmons, Klein and Simmons, 1977). This analysis focuses on the sets of norms that shape the feelings of living donors and recipients of kidney and bone marrow transplants. These rules are understood as normative obligations to give and receive. In this way the "gift of life" aspect of organ donation is analysed as an instance of the phenomenon of gift-exchange originally conceived in Mauss' The Gift (1954).

3. Some authors use the concept of sociotechnical systems (Burns and Flam, 1987:298-310). This consists, on the one hand, of complex technical structures which are designed to produce or to transform certain things, and, on the other, of social institutions and organisations designed to structure and regulate tasks/activities in which human agents are involved. The sub-structures may be owned or managed by different agents; the knowledge of these structures may be dispersed among different occupations and professions; different social networks, organisations, and institutions may be involved in the construction, operation and maintenance of substructures. In my work I

do not use the concept of sociotechnical systems but prefer to refer to the sociotechnical characteristics of the organisation.

4.   Another important sociological effort is the work of O'Neill in Australia (O'Neill, 1996).

5.   A tight-coupled process is a process that depends on small time marginal for its functioning (geographical to the same extent). This is particularly the case in OTS regarding the harvesting, extraction, preservation and implantation of the organs.

6.   The theory of sociotechnical systems provides a language and perspective for describing and analysing the organisation and development of a system such as the OTS (see among others, Emery and Trist, 1960; Herbst, 1974; Hughes, 1983; Mayntz and Hughes, 1988; Baumgartner and Burns, 1984; Burns and Flam, 1987; Andersen and Burns, 1990). In this theoretical perspective, the OTS can be characterised as a large-scale system with tight coupling and precise co-ordination of many types of actors, activities, and technologies (see also Joerges et al., 1990; Braun et al., 1991). It is a more or less clearly bounded system regulated by specific social rule systems, disposing of a specialised knowledge base, advanced technologies, specialised occupations and professions, and a high degree of internal relatedness (see Mayntz and Hughes, 1988; 1995b).

7.   This chapter is published in a different version in Human Systems Management, Vol. 11, 1992. Graphic work in the chapter has been made by Nicholas Burns. I am grateful to Anders Olsson for advice and encouragement in preparing the published version of this chapter.

8.   Brain death is established when the functions in cerebrum, cerebellum and brainstem irreversibly fail. Death criteria are non spontaneous respiration, no reflexes, no spontaneous movements, no responses to stimuli for 24 hours, electrocerebral silence.

9.   The OTS – its performance and development – depends on resources outside its total control (resources in its environment). The OTS – its designers and managers – develop strategic ties, exchange relations, etc. in order to gain access or some control over the strategic resources.

10.   The longer a patient waits for an organ in dialysis, the higher the chances of becoming immunised and rejecting a graft organ.

11.   With the development of more effective immunosuppression, the right tissue-matching between donor and recipient has lost some of its previous importance.

12.   This could eventually become an administrative vs. network tension if the demands on a centre – of competing for resources and clients – becomes critical. Also other tensions in exchange networks may arise (see Chapter 5).

13.   The medical personnel at the laboratories, as opposed to the transplantation unit, do not always agree whether to send away an organ or not. Even if the exchange rules are explicit, disagreements can arise about the applicability of the rule in particular cases. However, the transplantation centre is ultimately responsible and has the definitive decision. If the rules are not followed, the physician in charge must produce a legitimate explanation such as, e.g., a patient emergency.

14. This is the normal case for kidney transplantations where patients can be maintained in dialysis while they are waiting for the transplantation. Transplantations of hearts, lungs and livers are more often performed in conditions of emergency and frequently the patients are already at the hospital.

15. This structure may be subject to changes now, since later policies allow patients to choose freely any transplantation centre in the country independently of the assigned region (Rehn, 1994).

16. De facto organ transplantations are performed in Lund's lasarett. Conversely, organ transplantations are not performed at the moment in the Karolinska Hospital in Stockholm even if technically (officially) it is authorised to do so.

17. Other exceptions are experimental types of transplantations (brain tissue, etc.).

18. Additionally, the Scandinavian Transplantation Society stands for scientific cooperation between transplantation professionals.

19. The information also includes need of organs with particular characteristics, waiting time of patients in respective lists, expected outcomes, etc.

20. Repeated blood transfusions lead to patients becoming "sensitised", that is their immunity systems produce antibodies that react against several types of tissue. In order to increase the chances for these patients to retain a graft, they need an implant as close to their own tissue type as possible. In theory, the more a patient waits in, e.g., dialysis the more she/he becomes sensitised, making the task of finding a good match more difficult. This becomes a dilemma in the choice of recipients for transplantation (see Machado:1990).

21. The same surgeons can perform both the organ extraction and implantation of different organs, or some surgeons can be specialised in the extraction/implantation of particular organs, or less experienced surgeons may perform organ extractions, while the more experienced ones perform only implantations.

22. Initially the organ extraction was performed by local surgeons (where the donor was located) but currently the people of the transplantation team perform the extraction in order to improve the quality of the organ.

23. Access to an ICU is necessary for the care of operated patients but also as one of the sources of potential organ donors.

24. Eventually, potential donors can be treated at the thoracic, and children's ICU or at the emergency unit.

25. Often, relatives are present and even if a donation card is available, they are still informed and even consulted about an eventual donation (see also footnote 2).

26. The UAS transplantation unit signs the time reports of the extra personnel, and this automatically charges the costs to the T unit. No special forms or extra administrative work is used.

27. According to the law, blood circulation should not be maintained more than 24 hours after a person's death. Exceptionally this time can be extended (SOSFS 1987:32).

28. A kidney transplantation takes approximately 2-3 hours, and a liver transplantation 7-20 hours operation time.

29. The organisation of the Swedish transplantation system, with regional divisions, can be under a process of restructuration. It is not clear yet if the regions are to be maintained only for purposes of organ harvesting. Recent changes in the health care infrastructure support the development of a more flexible and market-oriented model. As a result of this there is a growing competition for better transplantation results but also a growing competition for patients (regardless of already established administrative regional divisions), and also for allocation of future professional technical or financial resources.

30. The transplantation centre is part of a hospital that also receives donors.

31. The organs procured come through different arrangements for the different centres. For example, in the Stockholm region most of the necroorgans come from the Neurosurgical Unit at the Karolinska Hospital which is not the location of transplantation activity in the region.

32. For reason of technical and ethical considerations, the donor body is never transported to the transplantation centre.

33. To specify all the key rules (actor rules, process rules and structure rules) governing the organisation of a transplantation system is beyond the scope of this work. Hence, I only provide illustrations of some key rules.

34. I have not dealt with processes on the structuration level (see Figures 4 and 5), which concern maintaining or changing the social rule regimes organising and regulating the transplantation process.

35. Other related laws are for example those laws referred to burials, etc. since they oversee the bodily integrity of the deceased and the will of the living. These laws are based on implicit or explicit concepts about human beings, their rights, their duties and proper behaviour (i.e. to vandalise graveyards is penalised by the law).

36. Ireland has no legal regulation of transplantation (up to 1995), but in practice consent from the deceased or his/her relatives is required. If the wishes of the deceased and relatives are in conflict, the opinion of the latter prevail. It is just the opposite in the practice of some countries, e.g. most Swiss cantons.

37. In May 1996 the Dutch Upper House ratified the law concerning organ donation stating that all Dutch citizens 18 years of age or older will be able to express their decision regarding organ donation in a central registry as a yes/no decision or the option of empowering the surviving next-of-kin or another person to make the decision. If no information is available the decision will be taken by surviving next-of-kin. Minors between 12 years and 16 years can also donate their organs but one of the parents can veto the decision. The registry became fully operational in 1988.

38. On June 25, 1997 the Deutscher Bundestag, the German federal parliament, approved a bill regulating organ transplants. Organs may be removed from a donor at the moment of confirmed brain death, by two independent physicians. Donation is regulated through a policy of non-presumed consent. In its absence, a relative or partner may give his or her consent, but may not oppose any known wishes of the donor. Regarding living donors, only a patient's close relatives or spouse may donate kidneys. The sale of organs has been banned.

39. A related issue concerns the legal determination of death. Most jurisdictions have specific provisions relating to the clinical condition for cadaveric organ donation (e.g. brain death) in their transplant statutes. But, the legal requirements for the certification of death vary widely. In Turkey death has to be established by four physicians not pertaining to the transplantation team. In Belgium, Greece, Hungary and Spain, death has to be established by three physicians not pertaining to the transplantation team. Italy requires three physicians, but the proscription of not pertaining to the transplantation team is omitted. In Bulgaria, France and Norway, the requirement is of two physicians not pertaining to the transplantation team. Romania allows the two physicians to be part of the transplantation team. In Denmark, Sweden, the Russian Federation and the United Kingdom, death can be certified solely by one physician, who cannot pertain to the transplantation team. Most laws explicitly state that disfigurement of the cadaver should be avoided.

40. However, there is considerable variation. For instance, the United Kingdom passed the Human Organ Transplant Act in 1989 in order to regulate the use of corpses for therapy and research. It states that authorisation from the person "in lawful possession of the body" is required in order to make use of a body. Since the legal agent can be an individual, e.g. a relative, or an institution (that is, the hospital), the law can be interpreted in practice as a form of presumed consent – but not explicitly.

41. Physicians tend to consider organ procurement a low priority among their pressing duties, particularly in large urban medical complexes (Dennis 1991: 19). Spain has introduced an organisational arrangement and an incentive system for carrying out the task of identifying potential donors and talking to and persuading next-of-kin. But the Spanish type system runs the risk of systematically violating the sensibilities of next-of-kin (and the integrity of the deceased citizen).

42. Historically, there has been a secular (modern) Western trend toward not only extending citizen rights to new categories of people (to all males, to women, children and people with disabilities) but also extending the rights of individuals vis-à-vis the state. The modern citizen is conceived legally as a rational agent, possessing rights to decide over certain things, physical property as well as over her own body. Twentieth-century legislation has strived to protect the right of private individuals to decide over their own bodies (Inger,1985). The period after World War Two can be characterised by a significant change of attitudes. The new attitudes were reflected in, for instance, the more careful decisions of the Swedish Board of Medicine regarding sterilisation of young individuals. Eugenic indications in medical case descriptions were replaced by medical indications. The decisive difference between the old sterilisation policy and the new genetic counselling was the shift from social to individual interest (Broberg and Tydén 1991:174). One of the first public expressions of this new attitude was articulated in Olof Palme's address to the Parliament in 1960 concerning the Sterilisation Act: "Societal right recedes on behalf of the individual right..." (quoted in Broberg and Tydén, 1991). There are few doubts that Swedish citizens have more to say about their bodies today than fifty years ago. For example, while in an official inquiry of 1936 the

notion of "a person deciding freely over her body" was characterised as a highly individualistic conception (SOU 1936:46:189), a follow up commissioned by the same organisation thirty years later established that "a person has in principle the right to decide over her body" (SOU: 1974:25). This trend towards increased individual rights was prevalent during the sixties, where several laws were amended decreasing the rights of the society to decide about the citizens' bodies. However, the expansion of individual rights over the body and its parts are under challenge today because of the rapid expansion of biotechnical developments. Biotechnical advances, for example gene-manipulation and organ transplantation, make the human body an extremely valuable object for research and therapy. Several expert debates and inquiries have centred about these questions, questions that concern the boundaries between individual rights on the one hand, and societal right and welfare (Michailkais, 1995; Brante and Hallberg, 1989). Simultaneously, the motif of the public good is prevalent in the mass media and public discourse concerning the importance of the new forms of treatment and research (i.e. the need of organs for transplantation). At the present, societal claims over human tissues and organs seem to have acquired greater legitimacy, and are taking prevalence over individual integrity by reason of the enormous usefulness of these body parts.

43. For those cases where the extraction of biological material would be required for medical purposes other than clinical transplantation (e.g. experimentation and fabrication of drugs), the law delegates the right to give authorisation to the Board of Health and Welfare (Transplant Act 1975:190).

44. In 1932 a decree (abolished 1973) regulated the uses of corpses for anatomical studies of individuals buried with the aid of public funds, those who died in mental hospitals, sanatoriums, prisons, and asylums (DsS 1974:5:81).

45. The transition from presumption of consent to non-presumed consent was in part connected to the introduction of new criteria for establishing death (see note 12), in part to ameliorate possible public suspicion or fear of organ harvesting and to assure the sustained legitimacy and authority of the medical profession. In addition, there was during the 1980s in Sweden a tendency to strengthen individual rights and integrity (Burns, 1995).

46. In 1987 legislation was passed defining total cerebral infarction as the criterion of death: the "Law about the Occurrence of Death". This law improved the performance of kidney transplants and opened up the possibility of performing heart transplantations in Sweden. The law does not in principle touch the question of rights. However, the law about death was understood by many to be closely connected to the Transplant Act, but they were dealt with separately in the preparation for the legislation and in the legislative process (Brante and Hallberg, 1989). Debates about the introduction of a legal criteria of death in Sweden started already in 1958 in connection with the first Transplant Act. Public and parliamentary controversies about whether or not to legislate a brain death concept went on for almost 30 years. Major concerns were the connection between brain death and opportunities for organ transplantation, questions about the reliability of determination of death by neurological criteria, a possible negative reaction

from the public in the turbulent 1970s, and the lack of parliamentary consensus. As one member of Parliament, former minister of Health, put it, "We do not want to give the public the impression that one party is for one type of concept of death and another party stands for another, that a change of political climate lead to changes in the constitutional laws. There have been diverse opinions inside the committee" (Michailakis, 1995). The timely solution began to take shape already in 1982, when the Minister of Health launched two separate governmental inquiries, one to analyse the pros and cons of legally establishing a criterion of death (eventually brain death), and the other inquiry to study eventual reforms of the Transplant Act. Each inquiry was carried out independently of the other. The Minister of Health was overtly explicit about this: the inquiry about eventual modifications to the current death criteria was to leave aside any considerations or consequences for transplantation. The rationale for this measure was explicitly formulated by a member of the Parliament: "We want to maintain a distinction between political decisions and medical decisions" (see Michailakis above). The issue was settled in 1987 when the brain death law was approved, by considering the cessation of the functions of the entire brain as equivalent to death. At that time, as discussed in the text, an amendment to the 1975 Transplantation Act was passed.

47. The concept of "public duty" that has characterised the Swedish legislation in these matters has to be understood in the context of the Swedish health care system, contrasting to the organisation of the USA health care that in the particular case of organ and tissue donations endorse a more "individualistic" transfer of "gifts of life" in its legislation, The Uniform Anatomical Gift Act of the USA Federal Legislation (1968,1987).

48. Necrodonation entails two very different legal circumstances in Sweden: direct donation takes place when the person herself expresses orally or in writing her wishes concerning the future uses of her body; proxy donation when a next-of-kin consents to donation. A direct donation entails few ambiguities on the question of individual autonomy, conforming closest to modern legal conceptions. A proxy donation takes place when – given a legal policy of non presumed consent – there is no written authorisation to organ extraction by the deceased, and the next-of-kin acts as (a) source of information giving evidence about the disposition of the deceased, or (b) as agent of the deceased and deciding in her/his place. Proxy donation conciliates the need of obtaining organs for transplantation and the legal requirement of obtaining a person's consent regarding actions on her body.

49. An amendment was introduced in 1988 stating that the physician must assure that the giver understands the implications of the procedure (SFS 1988:1275).

50. The opinion of children for medical procedures is generally taken into full consideration around puberty.

51. Next-of-kin: "someone that has been especially close to the deceased" (SOS:1989:98: 29, 158, 276). In practice the next-of-kin refers to the spouse, children, parents and siblings.

52. Since the higher mortality rates for men when compared to women is not accounted by higher incidences of disease but by accidents and trauma, these figures are expressions of a gendered pattern of risk behaviour. Thus in this very sense we can see the consequences of the social construction of gender.
53. Source: Transplant, Vol. 3, 1991, p. 173.
54. Source: Scandiatransplant.
55. Source: Scandiatransplant.
56. Source: Transplant, Vol. 4, 1992, p.107.
57. Source: Scandiatransplant.
58. Source: Scandiatransplant.
59. Source: Transplant, Vol. 3, 1991, p. 73.
60. Source: Transplant, Vol. 3, 1991, p. 47.
61. Source: Transplant, Vol. 4, 1992, p. 171.
62. Spain, England, Ireland and France show figures under 10% (Land and Dossetor, 1990).
63. Source: Fox and Sweazy, 1974:344.
64. Source: Dr. Dagfinn Ahlbrechtsen, Norwegian National Hospital, Oslo, Norway.
65. Source: Bunzendahl et al., 1991.
66. Source: Blohmé et al., 1992.
67. Source: Rowe, 1991.
68. Source: Alexolopolus et al., 1991.
69. Source: Simforoosh et al., 1991.
70. Source: Sutherland et al., 1991.
71. Source: Sutherland et al., 1991.
72. Source: Francis et al., 1992.
73. Source: Whitington et al., 1991.
74. Source: Whitington et al., 1991.
75. The concept of altruism has been discussed not only in relation to individual actions but also in connection with welfare policies, e.g. blood or organ donation. The access to blood is imperative to any sizeable hospital; organ transplantation depends on access to human biological material, many research programs depend on access to experimental subjects and to corpses. The opinions about which are the most effective and morally right policies for obtaining, for example, blood and organs are varied and conflicting.
76. This "sacrifice" does not necessarily have to respond to generalised notions of rightness or morality. There are references to individuals willing to donate their hearts or lungs while alive for the expressed purpose of helping others.
77. Less straightforward forms of payment are the "incentives" to donation such as tax refunds or payment of funerals of the deceased (Davis, 1989).
78. The rules of social exchange in, e. g., a family can be more or less strained depending on the characteristic of the donation. Giving renewable tissue does not entail the seriousness of giving solid organs, and the particular configuration of the network of rights and duties in each family determines the willingness or not to donate. For

example, the configuration "mother giving to daughter or son" is the strongest socially prescribed form of giving in the family network, together with "husband gives to wife and vice versa". When the donation pattern in a family follows this line, it is consistent with the stipulated social norm and the potential conflict of interest minimal. In other cases, e.g.: "brother to sister", the social norms of rights (giving) and duties are more unconstrained and do not legitimise the donation of the organ to the same extent.

79. In donating one's own body parts after death the temporal distance is infinite since the actor will never experience the actualisation of his/her action.

80. In a certain sense sacrifice is regarded as synonymous to altruism in August Comte's meaning. The concept of altruism was coined by Comte as the key term in the "civil religion" he conceived and that would have the function of ennobling the citizens and internalise their beliefs in the the good society, its objective and future (in contrast to Rousseau, he does not attach supernatural or logical references to it, his moral concepts are based on more purely social dimensions). While his Positive Scientific system (sociological) stood for order, the civil religious system stood for progress (as a necessary latent substratum for the scientific system – that alone could not sustain the necessary moral cohesion in society). The individual in Comte's conception was conceptualised as an abstraction representing social and cultural traits.

81. The bio-chemical factors that differentiate individuals and are responsible for graft rejects are called antigens. One example is the well-known blood cell classification into groups. Blood type (O, A, B, AB) compatibility and incompatibility operate in the following way (Punch, 1998). Blood cells have particular proteins. A person's immunological system reacts against incompatible proteins. If a patient receives an organ that has incompatible proteins on it, for example A proteins in the case of a B type patient, the organ will fail quickly, within minutes. A B type person will naturally have antibodies against A type proteins. For reasons of fairness, organs may be allocated primarily to their own blood group. Otherwise, the O patients, who are universal donors but can only accept O organs, would only have access to a fraction of the organs, while AB patients would have access to all organs. Even with re-allocation rules, there are inequities in the waiting times of particular blood group lists. This explains why there are often rules readjusting and biasing blood type patients access to kidneys in the interest of equity.

   In the case of liver, heart, and lung transplants, "matching" is generally not conducted except for blood group (O, A, B, AB) and organ size. For instance, in the case of livers, it is known that one can even use blood group incompatible livers (an A liver in a B patient) with success rates almost as good as blood group identical livers. Why this is so is not clear (Punch, 1998).

82. Besides the red blood cell classification into groups, another system of inherited white blood cell groups, distinct from the red cell groups. There are several genetic markers located on the surface of most of our white cells. One particular group of genetic markets is called Human Leukocyte Antigens (leukocyte refers to white cell, and antigen refers to genetic marker) or HLA. Tissue typing is the name given to the test

which identifies an individual's HLA. This information is to a greater or lesser extent critical in determining if a patient should be implanted with a particular organ (Punch, 1998). If two persons have exactly the same HLA, they are "identical matches", for instance two siblings. Or two siblings may share one plus half of the same HLA, which is referred to as "one-haplotype match". If there is no sharing of HLA, this is referred to as "two-haplotype mismatch". An individual's tissue type can thus be defined and compared to those of potential donors. The relevance of tissue typing to kidney graft results has been demonstrated in intrafamilal transplantation, but also accumulated experience with implanting kidneys with varying degrees of match with the recipient.

In addition to tissue type, there is a second test, the "crossmatch", which indicates if there is specific immune reactivity between donor and recipient (Punch, 1998). The crossmatch is performed by mixing a very small amount of the patient's serum with a very small amount of the potential donor's white cells (where the HLA are on the surface of the white cells) to determine if a reaction will take place. If the patient has antibodies (proteins), the donor's cells will be injured. This is referred to as a "positive crossmatch". Such a crossmatch is a contraindication to transplant since it signifies that the patient has the ability to destroy the donor's cells, and would most likely destroy the donor's implanted kidney. A negative crossmatch indicates the patient does not have the HLA antibody against that particular donor, and a transplant can be performed. In general, if a patient receives a mismatched kidney, it will not function and be promptly rejected (by antibodies action).

83. There are six categories of HLA (designated by the letters HLA-A, -B, -C, -DP, -DQ, -DR) with sub-groupings within each category (O'Neill, 1996:52). Patients awaiting a transplant are tested to determine their tissue type. Such information is included with other information about patients on a waiting list. An ideal recipient would match on all six categories of HLAs. In some allocation systems, matching is given priority over other criteria, or given substantial points in a "point system". If perfect matching is not obtained, then one looks for a potential recipient with four HLA matches.

84. France Transplant uses the following rules for national distribution (Dennis et al., 1991:10): If there is a perfectly matched candidate or a sensitised patient having at least a five-antigen match with the donor, the kidney is shared. If there is not a suitable recipient on the national list, allocative rights revert to the Regional office within which the procuring transplant team operates; each regional office of France Transplant has a waiting list stratified by ABO blood type, according to quality of HLA match.

85. Eurotransplant is an international foundation with the transplant centres of the member countries represented. After discussion of an issue or policy proposal in special advisory committees and in the General Assembly (with representatives of all the centres), decisions are taken by the Eurotransplant Board, where all member countries are represented. For instance, after extensive preparations and discussions with Eurotransplant, the Eurotransplant Board decided on January 17, 1996 to introduce a new allocation system (X-COMB), a computer program or algorithm, for kidneys.

86. That is type O kidneys are transplanted only in type O or type B transplant candidates;

type A in A, AB; B in B, AB; and AB in AB.

87. The factor "Mismatch Probability" is an estimate of the probability of a kidney offer with 0 and 1 broad HLA-A, B, DR antigen mismatch from 1000 kidneys offered, taking into account the ABO blood group matching rules and the percentage of the latest PRA screening. The factor is a multiplication of three terms: 0 or 1 HLA mismatch probability, ABO blood group and PRA screening.

88. This factor distinguishes 5 levels of distance with the points indicated in parentheses: local (300), equivalent (a collaborative group of transplant centres)(300), regional (208), national (104), international (0). If the transplant candidate has his/her residence outside the Eurotransplant area, no points are assigned.

89. The formula here is:

Score = 200 x (waiting time of the transplant candidate in days) ÷ 2191.

That is, all transplant candidates who have been waiting 6 years (2191 days) receive the maximum of 200 points.

90. This factor concerns for each member country of Eurotransplant, the net exchange between itself and all the other countries. "Export" is a net negative exchange: the number of kidney transplants performed in the country is less than the number of kidneys procured. "Import" occurs when the number of kidneys procured is less than the number of kidney transplants performed. The balance is then positive. If the candidate has his/her residence outside the Eurotransplant area, no points are assigned.

91. The formula to assign points for the factor "HLA-antigen mismatch" is based on the number of mismatches on the loci HLA-A, HLA-B and HLA-DR: Score = 400 x (1 - (sum of broad HLA-A, B, DR antigen mismatches ÷ 6)). As pointed earlier, an HLA-antigen mismatch occurs when a donor HLA-antigen would be recognised by the recipient as being different from the recipient's own HLA-antigens.

92. The rule for highly immunised patients is complex. There is a default clause stating that if a preliminary cross-match – to be performed at the tissue typing laboratory, associated with the donor centre – is negative, a kidney will be offered. In case the result of the preliminary cross-match is positive or in case it is impossible to perform a cross-match, regardless of the underlying cause (no serum of the patient present, no capacity), no kidney offer will be made to the immunised patient.

93. Another type of default rule concerns the response of transplant centre to an offer of a kidney for one of its patients. Directly after a firm offer has been made. The transplant centre has to communicate its decision on the kidney offer within 60 minutes from the time of offering. If the centre has not replied within 60 minutes, Eurotransplant may skip the priority of the transplant centre involved and upgrade the centre of the next patient on the list. After making an initial offer decision, Eurotransplant, as a backup measure, approaches other transplant centres with a provisional kidney offer (back-up offer). If a transplant centre declines a firm offer, the first-back-up offer becomes a firm offer.

Again, even other types of problems are defined and their solutions formally specified. For example, if a kidney transplant program informs the officers on duty at

Eurotransplant, after the receipt of a kidney, that the kidney cannot be transplanted in the patient for whom they have accepted they kidney, the officers (in consultation with the medical staff at Eurotransplant) decide whether the kidney can be transplanted at the same transplant program into any (other) back-up recipient. Of course, this will depend on the presence of other suitable recipients, presently on the allocation list, taking into account the already passed cold ischemia time and need for cross-matching.

94. Australia is another type of decentralised system in each of the six states (O'Neill, personal communication, 16.4.97). Kidneys are allocated on the basis of matching of HLAs. The best match is allocated the kidney. If no "perfect" match (a match on all six types of HLAs) then the organ is allocated to the next best match (this could be a match on five, four or three HLAs). If there are two or more recipients with equivalent HLA matches, then the organ is allocated to the patient who has been on dialysis for the longest period.

95. Sixty-six organ procurement organisations (since the early 1990s) exist in the USA. A total of more than 20,360 organ transplants were performed in 1996 (of these 8598 being kidneys). As many as 40,000 individuals needing transplants are waiting for organs. The United Network for Organ Sharing [UNOS] is a nationally organised organ allocation system. OPOs administer organ donation programs and co-ordinate the local procurement and distribution of necro-kidneys and other solid organs (hearts, lungs, livers and pancreas). The OPOs are nodes of the federally mandated Organ Procurement and Transplantation Network. The Network is operated by the UNOS; it maintains the national registry of patients awaiting organ transplantation. Since 1987 kidneys have been distributed according to a point system designed by UNOS. All distributions are made according to an algorithm operating with point scores for six different factors (see below). All transplant candidates are registered on one or more lists (see discussion in text).

UNOS operates with the following factors: (1) waiting time; (2) quality of antigen mismatch; (3) panel reactive antibody; (4) medical urgency; (5) paediatric status; and (6) donor status. Total points are calculated, as indicated below, for candidates who have ABO blood types compatible with that of the donor and who are active on the UNOS Patient Waiting List.

(1) Time of Waiting. Candidates may be assigned points for absolute as well as relative waiting times. For each full year of waiting time, a patient accrues 1 point. There are separate calculations for each geographic (local, regional and national) level of kidney allocation. The local points calculation includes only patients on the local Patient Waiting List. The regional calculation includes only patients on the regional list, without the local patients. The national points calculation includes all patients on the national list excluding all patients listed on the Host OPO's local and regional lists. A point is assigned to the patient waiting for the longest period with fractions of points being assigned proportionately to all other patients, according to their relative times of waiting. For instance, if there are 100 persons of O blood type waiting for kidneys, the person waiting the longest would receive 1 point (100/100 x 1 = 1). The next person in

order would receive a fraction of one point defined by the following equation: 99/100 x 1 = .99.

(2) Quality of Antigen Mismatch. A zero antigen mismatch is defined as occurring when a patient has an ABO blood type that is compatible with that of the donor and the patient and donor both have all six of the same HLA-A, B, and DR antigens. Points are thus assigned to a patient based on the number of mismatches between the patient's antigens and the donor's antigens: 7 points are assigned if there are no B or DR mismatches; 5 points if there is 1 B or DR mismatched, and 2 points if there is a total of 2 mismatches of the B and DR loci, etc.

UNOS has an elaborate complex of rules for allocating kidneys in the case where two or more patients have identical blood type, zero antigen mismatch with a donor. For example, if the patients are local, then select the one(s) with phenotypic identity between donor and patient. Then take another of the local patients. Continuing: select among those 80% or higher PRA patients on the list of OPOs which are owed a payback kidney, in the case that there is phenotypic identity between donor and patient, etc. until one comes to the national list.

(3) Panel Reactive Antibody. A patient is assigned 4 points if he or she has a panel reactive antibody (PRA) level of 80% or greater and there is a negative preliminary crossmatch between the donor and that patient.

(4) Medical Urgency. Locally, the patient's physician has the authority to use medical judgement in assignment of medical urgency points if there is only one renal transplant centre. When there is more than one local renal transplant centre, a co-operative medical decision is required prior to assignment of medical urgency points. No points are assigned to patients based upon medical urgency for regional or national allocation of kidneys.

(5) Paediatric Status. Kidney transplant candidates who are less than 11 years old are assigned four additional points for kidney allocation. Candidates who are 11 years old or older but less than 18 years old are assigned three additional points for kidney allocation. These points are assigned when the candidate is registered on the UNOS Patient Waiting List and retained until the candidate reaches 18 years of age.

(6) Donor Status. A patient is given 4 points if he or she has donated for transplantation his or her vital organ or a segment of a vital organ (that is, kidney, liver segment, lung segment, partial pancreas, small bowel segment).

96. Even if the Swedish Transplants Act regulates organ donation and the hospital regulations are of national character, there are no explicit general rules regulating the allocation of organs. The constant medical and technological developments of the field, are one of the most common reasons given for this lack of formalised rules of allocation. However, there is a general consensus about key criteria – among the nephrologists and dialysis physicians of a transplantation region associated with transplantation in the area studied, criteria established and reinforced by frequent contacts with the transplantation centre (visits of the regional transplantation co-ordinator to the donor hospital, seasonal meetings). The guidelines applied in the prioritisation and selection of patients for

transplantation indicate some variation between centres, but the general premises are similar.

97. UNOS refers to four categories of medical criteria: (1) anatomical and immunological compatibility of the donor and recipient; (2) medical urgency; (3) efficiency in physically moving the organ from the donor to the recipient in a way that ensures organ viability and improves the chances of a successful transplant; and (4) medical ethical considerations.

98. For example, a transplanted patient has to be aware of facts such as that a common cold can eventually provoke a powerful immunological reaction of the graft organ.

99. Other criteria more refer to infrastructural conditions: for example, location of the cadaver donor, a practical criteria determined by the extent of the geographical area to cover and the possibilities of a minimum preservation of the organ; patient access to adequate post-transplantational medical controls. These criteria are generally not relevant in a country like Sweden, a country of medium size and with well equipped local hospitals and excellent transportation networks.

100. The focus on compatibility criteria as a major basis for classifying recipients makes medical sense. It is not arbitrary or unwarranted. Similarly, the use of criteria relating to hyper-immunity make medical sense, and therefore appear fair.

101. In general, there is widespread awareness of the dilemma of local need and global demand, and formulate local and non-local distribution protocols. Many believe that decentralised kidney distribution increases the supply of organs. Under Scandiatransplant, a centre keeps one kidney and shares the other. France also operates according to the principle, "keep one, share one". The shared kidney is distributed according to an explicit protocol by French Transplant (the Etablissement Français des Greffes has taken over this function today).

102. The UNOS, as a result of the National Transplants Act of 1984, is administered under the Health Resources and Service Administration. According to its standards, transplant centres are subject to review if their survival rates for organ transplantation are in the lowest 5%. Full approval requires 12 cases/year and a minimum survival rate of 73 percent at 1 year and 65 percent at 2 years (Surman, 1989).

103. A key principle underlying the analysis is that rule, systems are not orderly logical structures, but are the result of historical and social processes in specific contexts, where the actors involved, enact, interpret and re-define those rules. This principle can be referred to as the Principle of Piecemeal Rule Formation and Development.

104. The history of the development of complex sociotechnical systems (such as OTS) suggests that social organisational and political problems are as much a challenge as the purely technical (Baumgartner and Burns, 1984; Burns and Flam, 1987; Burns and Ubehorst, 1988).

105. Two main types of roles and role relationships can be distinguished between patients and physician in hospital settings: (a) non-voluntary: special patient categories strictly subject to authorities and control on a regular basis: for example the mentally ill and children. These patients do not have the right to decide whether or not to participate; (b)

voluntary: the individual decides to participate or not. If the choice is "yes", she participates under conditions that are not of her making. In particular, she submits herself to the authority and rule order of the hospital. I regard both voluntary and non-voluntary relationships in hospital settings as formal and hierarchical.

106. There are official guidelines for how the Swedish Health Care Act and hospital regulations are to be interpreted and implemented.

107. The patient-physician relationship comprises several aspects. The one chosen as central to the analysis here is the formal-hierarchical one, i.e. administrative, where transplantation patients are in a sense part of the social organisation. "Patients" in hospital organisations can be defined as units in a health production process where the patients' roles could be situated in a continuum, from "patient" as passive recipient or the object of a health production process in one extreme, and "patient" as active part of that process in the other. The first pole will be emphasising patient as object/client, and the second pole will be emphasising patient as team-member/client (Anbäcken, 1985:10). Consequently, the first patient type would be regarded as external to the production process (but as the object of that process instead), and the second as internal to the health production process (administratively regulated). In specialised surgery such as transplantation, patients not only have to submit themselves to the "total institution" routines of the hospital (e.g. hospital eating hours, hospital clothes, waiting for the "round" to see a physician, etc.), but also after receiving a transplant, these patients have to follow detailed medical indications and controls (some of them all their life) in order to avoid organ rejection. In accepting (and carrying out) the directives of the physicians, these patients participate in the transplantation process, becoming an active and integral part of a health production process that is basically administratively regulated. In principle, noncompliant attitudes could imply the patient being removed as possible candidate for a transplant (an uncooperative patient that does not follow medical instructions could jeopardise an expensive operation and a donated organ would be wasted). Furthermore, according to the Swedish legal system, the relationship between patients and national health care is not contractual but administratively regulated (Rynning, 1994).

108. One might view market as the opposite of an "organisation" (read administration), but increasingly markets are being considered within the sociology of organisations (Burns and Flam, 1987; Ouchi, 1980; Thompson et al., 1991). Ouchi (1980) stresses that a market is as much a social organisation as a bureaucracy or a clan.

109. For example, by cultural conceptions about what is constituted as a marketable article; by political or moral considerations, etc.

110. There is an implicit reciprocal contract. The hospital does not have the right to do whatever they want with the body or body parts, e.g. to use them in education.

111. Studies about the power structure in the medical profession pointed at the existence of formal and informal relationships between colleagues, the formal related to superior or subordinate positions in medical institutions, and the informal related to interpersonal professional linkages (e.g. informal definitions of the quality of each other's work and

personal characteristics). Both studies indicated that position, status and power became recognised and perpetuated within the profession through formal and informal ways (Cockerham, 1978: 136). Thus professions can be understood as not only as formal associations coupled to administration but also as networks. Professional networks include hierarchical (status oriented: e.g. relationship of advisor and adequate discussion partners) as well as egalitarian (e.g. collegial and friendship) informal relationships (Coleman, et al., 1957:266). Network relationships seem to be activated in uncertain situations (Coleman et al., 1957:269).

112. Other sources of complexity are diversity of technologies (Joerges, 1988) and the number of different specialities (or division of labour) (Alter and Hage, 1993).

113. Since professional networks concern professional relationships, they comprise a limited segment of possible social relationships.

114. These are cognitive frames that specify which aspects of a situation are to be considered as relevant facts in understanding a situation (Anspach, 1993).

115. As an illustration of a not-uncommon situation, Professor M. Yacoub at the Old Court Hospital in London, during an interview, complained that the hospital had not received a single heart from Sweden, in spite of the fact that between 1988 and 1990, about ten Swedish patients were on the English waiting lists for heart transplants (Expressen, 1990).

116. The classification of organisational rule systems in the analysis is not based on empirical estimates but on the principle that it is in the pattern of co-ordinating rules that the "nature" of a social organisation is found.

117. Fox points out (1988:429) that the nurses and physicians who care for dying patients need special defences and supports to help them maintain "detached concern" in situations that normally arouse the deepest kind of anxiety and questioning about human suffering and mortality.

118. Perrow (1979) and Cockerham (1978) have stressed that relationships organised on a professional basis can generate tensions if combined with bureaucratic relationships within the same organisation or unit (Parsons, 1964). Thus, an individual may be the administrative supervisor (bureaucratic authority) of another with a higher professional competence but still under the authority of the former. This kind of organisational incongruity is typical of hospitals as examples of professional bureaucracies, and a frequent source of tensions and conflicts.

119. Application of one set of criteria would simplify the choice and worsen its results, since it would not account for the variation between cases.

120. The notion of integrative processes is found in Alter and Hage (1993), Etzioni (1975), Haas and Drabek (1973), Lawrence and Lorsch (1967), and, of course, Parsons (1961), among others. Our conception extends the range of mechanisms, including such devices as organisational ritual, non-task-oriented discourses, the role of humour and denigration, the spacing and architecture of organisations as well as mediating or buffering roles and institutional arrangements that minimise tensions and conflicts.

121. Scott (1981) deals with a variety of mediating relationships and positions, consideration

of which would take us beyond the scope of this chapter: contracting, sub-contracting, joint ventures, associations, informal linkages and networks.

122. During the time where the Harvard commission prepared the model for the new brain-death criteria – the 1960s – the social situation in the USA was one of a general distrust of experts, popular suspicion about "heroic" medicine (and that organs were taken from dying individuals), increasing public concern about the possibility of "living vegetables" maintained in the hospitals for years also indirectly creating legal problems of heritage, and a socially accepted criterion that bodies can be cremated. The medical viability of organs for transplants has already been proven and created a demand for "biologically living organs and dead organisms" (Everett Mendelsohn, lecture given at the Swedish Collegium for Advanced Study in the Social Sciences, Uppsala, Sweden, 1995).

123. Brain-related criteria revolve around 3 kinds of observations: The first is clinical observation of an absence of certain brain functions, e.g. shining a light in the eye and observing no pupil response, or putting ice water in the ear and observing no eye movement. Another entails the use of an electroencephalogram, commonly known as an EEG, but this is not mandatory in many protocols and legislation. The EEG is a recording of electrical activity from the surface of the brain. Angiography, a method to measure circulation of blood in the brain, is sometimes used. Prange (in Machado, 1990) refers to the degree of reliability of a number of technical investigations for the confirmation of brain-death. Fifty consecutive patients with suspected brain-death were included in his study to evaluate the reliability of different diagnostic techniques. The techniques employed comprised clinical examination, apnoea testing, EEG, extracranial Doppler ultrasonography (ECD), brainstem acoustic evoked potentials (BAEP) and arterial digital subtraction angiography (DSA). In 39 cases he reports no discrepancies in the results of the different techniques used to determine or confirm brain-death. With the remaining 11 cases the findings were not exactly concordant or, at least, permitted varying interpretations. For example, in six cases doubts existed as to whether or not the EEG was isoelectric (i.e., having or representing zero difference of electric potential). In four patients BAEP findings were compatible with brain-death two to three days before intracranial circulatory arrest was documented. Finally, in two patients with isoelectric EEG and absent BAEP, arterial DSA showed residual cerebral flow (Machado, 1992).

124. In the USA, the strategies developed in order to cover the demand for organs are the obligatory request for organ donation to the personnel, the creation of independent organ procurement agencies, appealing to the public in the media and lately the use of NHBDs (non heart beating donors). The most common methods adopted in the European countries to increase the organ supply is to circumvent the problem through the implementation of "presumed consent" policies, launching "awareness campaigns" highlighting the need for organs and reorganising the system of organ harvesting.

125. This model above is an instance of a more general problem concerning multiple concrete processes of social construction, the possible contradiction among these and their possible integration.

126. This model has to be understood as representing a phase in the reconstruction of the

body. The same process in a larger perspective is not linear, and includes feedback and loops not considered here.

127. In this chapter I do not deal with the issue of the role of rituals in health care and the disruption of those rituals in, for instance, intensive care units (see Chapter 8).

128. There is however a scientific controversy internal to the profession about where to establish decisive criteria (whether lower brain stem or higher brain failure) and about the accuracy of "brain-death" certification.

129. The use of NHBD (non heart beating donors), as a way of solving the problem of organ scarcity, it is to my knowledge still limited to some centres in the world. The NHBDs appear as a new category of corpse.

130. Veatch claims that the criteria of "whole brain-death" to certify death is unclear, that its advocates drew a somehow arbitrary line while advocates of the higher brain definition draw another line. Given the character of process that transition between death and life has, doubts and dissonances seem to be intrinsic to the application of whatever criteria chosen (Veatch, 1993a).

131. There are two broad classes of cognitive primary frames in Western societies for classifying phenomena, the "natural" and the "social" (Goffman, 1974). The natural frame is characterised by the (natural) event, "the natural course of things". It is a more mechanistic and deterministic understanding of events (determined by natural forces). In a social frame the concept of event is replaced by the deed, caused by human or suprahuman action implying agency, motivations and meanings (Goffman,1974).

132. A braindead body sustained by a respirator does not exhibit obvious differences from a living but comatose patient.

133. Phenomena or events understood as culturally misplaced, i.e. outside established cultural categories, become frightening. For example, corpses improperly buried are "unsettled" and may become "wandering souls" as a result.

134. Most transplantation centres take precautions to safeguard the identity of the donors' respective organ receivers.

135. Even more complex distinctions appear for example in the categorisation of immature foetuses.

136. The importance attributed to agency in the certification of death (i.e., braindead) is expressed in the laws and regulations for organ transplantation in most countries, requiring that the certification of brain-death will not be performed by the same physician responsible for transplantation patients. The purpose of these legal rules is to disengage the certification of death from any other concerns than benefit to the patient in the intensive care units. Initially, the concerns referred to in these laws were, for example, other patients' need of organs, but more recent developments threat to blur the line. There is a stage at which the mere prolongation of body function is no longer clearly worthwhile (i.e. "futility of treatment"), but a decision to avoid further life-saving measures depends not only on a medico-technical decision but also on the patient's advanced directives – or their family. Thus, the line that separates the moral and technical aspects of medicine in these decisions becomes thinner and thinner, in

other words facts and values, event and deed (Toulmin, 1990). Regarding the personnel at the intensive care and emergency units, legal measures have been, for example, obligatory request, the establishment of OPOs, and intensive information and campaigns.

137. The time limit for a braindead to be maintained has successively increased from "some hours or days", to "few weeks" to "a few months" in latter cases (apparently well over a year for children). In other words, even if brain-death is an intermediate stadium, it can be maintained for a considerable amount of time. The factor that apparently influences this development is the increased medical and nursing investment in the maintenance of these braindead.

138. This and the following chapter are based on collaborative work with Tom R. Burns.

139. "Denial of death" is often given a psychological explanation, the individual's inherent fear or anguish in the face of death (Sanner, 1991). While there is certainly some truth in this, an alternative hypothesis stemming from our theory is that "denial of death", in general terms, is the result of a rupture or destabilisation of a given cognitive and emotional frame (Goffman (1974) speaks in general about the "vulnerability of perceptual frames"). In the particular case of dealing with the braindead, it is the result of a fracture produced by rule frame incompatibility and conflict, not by vague notions of the psychological frailty of individuals (in which of course particular cases may play some role).

140. Festinger's theory of cognitive dissonance has been an influential theory in the field of psychology. It resulted in considerable research, giving new insight into otherwise incomprehensible human behaviour. For example, why we grow to like things which we suffer from (Aronson and Mills, 1959); why we came to despise an innocent victim of our abuse (Davis and Jones, 1960); how can our beliefs change as a result of misleading another person (e.g. Festinger and Carlsmith, 1959); how mild threats to punishment can lead to greater compliance than harsh threats (Aronson and Carlsmith, 1963; Freedman, 1965), and so on (see Thibodeau and Aronson, 1992).

141. It is not possible in this limited chapter to provide an adequate review of the extensive literature on cognitive balance theories, including the substantial contributions of the theory of cognitive dissonance.

142. Since the 50's the original postulates have been revised and criticised on several premises. Among the more important developments of this theory in psychology are the following: inconsistent cognitions alone are not enough to produce dissonance, without considering the critical role of behavioural commitment (Brem and Cohen, 1962); the role of individuals' self-concept is central in mediating dissonance (Aronson, 1968; Thibodeau and Aronson, 1992); the sense of personal responsibility is an important ingredient in dissonance experiences (Brehm and Wicklund, 1976). However, the fundamental postulates remain unchanged.

143. A number of states of "patient passivity" are distinguished. That is, there is an elaborate category system – as is typical of important areas of action (recall the story of Eskimos distinguishing many different types of snow). The distinctions may not only be made for

medical reasons – that is, what types of treatment called for – but also for legal or administrative reasons: what can and cannot be done with the patient; what should or must be done under certain circumstances. There are also moral aspects that play a role in the distinctions.

144. Cognitive consistency is no ultimate goal or value. As Billig et al. (1988) have argued, actors live with and accept many inconsistencies.

145. The rule systems, and in particular the values and norms that apply, and the ways in which actors are to morally and emotionally orient themselves will then differ in the two situations.

146. This proposition stresses the structural bases of major dissonance experiences. Otherwise as Billig (1982) and Billig et al. (1988) suggest, people frequently experience dissonance without serious consequences.

147. Taking into consideration variances in what is regarded as a tolerable level of ambiguity or uncertainty (that is defined as inconsequential and can be set aside), a certain dose of ambiguity is contingent to most organisational situations. This level of uncertainty is defined by the organisational norms that establish the boundaries or limits of tolerability.

148. Another type of strategy is to seek assent (approval, support) for a decision already made within the medical group, for example when making the decision to discontinue treatment (Anspach, 1993).

149. It is not in the scope of this work to investigate the differential power and status of doctors and nurses within the medical order, although this is a significant factor. Moreover, there is an obvious gender aspect as well in that the dominant profession is made up mostly of men and the dominated profession is made up mostly of women.

150. Collective representations and classificatory systems – and the collective cognitive-normative frames of which they are a part – are social facts, and in an historical perspective, social constructions.

151. Billig et al. (1988) would probably refer to these as ideologies.

152. An often mentioned issue relating to organ procurement is people's poor knowledge about the nature of "brain death". Most people tend to associate death with a motionless cold body, a "lifeless" body, in other words, death is identified with lack of bodily vital symptoms. But, in fact, braindead patients whose circulatory functions are sustained are warm and pink.

153. Patients with severe brain damage are often put into deep sedation in order to help the recovery.

154. A series of confirmatory tests are available, such as brain scanning etc.

155. The conception of brain death is generally accepted but there continues to be controversy about whether or not cortical death is sufficient as brain death criteria.

156. As in Festinger et al. (1956), people act on this judgement; they committed themselves to radical changes in their lives.

157. This relates to belief in the physician's words that somebody that breathes in the ventilator is dead, and of the two ways of reasoning (analytical and contextual-

emotional), also the role of incorporating a new view.

158. Anspach (1993:50) arrives at similar conclusions about the organisational basis of prognostic judgement, in a study about decision-making in nurseries for premature infants. Physicians, nurses and "parents" are actor categories that differ in their access to information, resources and power, and each group shares commonalties of interest and are bearers of particular subcultures.

159. As pointed out somewhere else in the chapter, the normative and knowledge bases are different for different types of professional, service-oriented organisations.

160. Douglas (1987) suggests that true solidarity in groups and organisations is based on such shared classifications and collective representations. Moreover, collectives experience crisis – a deep sense of disorder and chaos – in the absence of, or a loss of confidence in their, collectively shared and individually internalised classification schemes.

161. Shared values specify what is desirable or undesirable, assigning values to objects, agents, actions, events, states of the world, and developments, which are classified and differentially evaluated in the particular social order. That is, these concern those things which should be valued, pursued, or at least pursued in a particular institutional domain or set of relationships. Such rules also indicate what should be avoided or destroyed as "evil", what are the "right ways to do things" (Burns and Flam, 1987).

162. Weick (1979) recognises the problem of social order, and the need of actors who try to maintain an order to reduce through coding and classification disturbances (exclusion of information, persons, and materials; or proper routeing of them). At the same time, the organisation must be open enough to learn from and to adapt to its environment, which is changing. That is, to find a balance between stability and change.

163. Anspach (1993) stresses the importance of correctly classifying, e.g. in terms of what the problem is and thus how it ought to be handled. This is obvious in the case of dead or not dead, where the question has legal and even criminal implications.

164. As suggested earlier, organisational rituals and discourses play an important role in the maintenance of boundaries between social/medical categories and in orderly changes of status (passages).

165. Even groups of low status, low authority groups, may be reluctant to give up an established collective identity (even as they may aspire to change their identity and status). With such a definition, they have established strategies, are predictable for themselves and for others.

166. As indicated earlier, I am assuming that actions have been taken, events have occurred – there is a fait accompli. In many instances, professionals have opportunities to correct "mistakes" or to modify their behaviour. In general, actors in their various roles and positions, e.g. those responsible for the clinic or hospital, physicians or nurses, try to behave in ways consistent with their identities – to maintain their image or presentation of self – consistent with their identities. In part, they try to avoid or reduce incongruence between identity standards (commitments) and their actions (or at least perceptions and judgements of their actions).

167. Complex social organisations give rise to contradictions, ambiguities, confusion, disorder, conflict and struggle because of the heterogeneous and contradictory social relationships and institutional arrangements that make up complex social organisation (see Chapter 5). The juxtapositions and interfacing of different principles and modes of organising imply that actors involved in any given organising mode or institutional order experience signals, events, developments which are dissonance producing. And those involved utilise discourses, rituals, as well as more obvious instrumental strategies to help maintain collective representations – and the basis of social order – for example, in terms of the global frame of modern medicine that key professional groups are competent and trustworthy, that any particular action can be explained and justified in these terms.

168. Individual and collectively shared conceptions and interpretations of core elements in the cognitive-normative frame, and their realisation in practices, may diverge. Innovators and entrepreneurs are often deviants.

169. Some disturbances, challenges, or conflicts disrupt or threaten to disrupt the hospital order more than others, for example important outside authorities or powerful interests may precipitate crises, by questioning or challenging medical authority, medical practices. Or conflicts which arise within the medical staff, especially between groups of physicians, are highly disruptive, much more disruptive than conflict between staff and next-of-kin, because they undermine or threaten to undermine the legitimacy of the medical order as a scientific order, a source of solid and reliable knowledge and an institution dedicated as a whole to serving its clients.

170. Orders tend to operate so as to keep authoritative or powerful outsiders from challenging the order. This is critical. Thus, medical or legal experts outside the hospital may obtain data or results and make judgements which are authoritative, legitimate, or so powerful that normal internal mechanisms of dissonance reduction are not likely to work. One way this takes place in the USA is through legal processes of challenging medical orders and their key agents. These may have several paths: (1) professionals or parents can turn to the courts or authorities when they disagree with a judgement, decision, or handling in a hospital; (2) someone in the staff itself may disagree with the decision and report the case to government agencies; (3) the mass media or a political group may learn of an action or decision and appeal to authorities to take action, or may simply report it to the press. (Anspach stresses that encounters with the legal system are rare, but they are substantial economic and professional threats.)

171. Initiatives from within entail adopting or developing a new perspective, new value orientations, introduction of new technologies or techniques, which generate or lead to quite new types of ambiguities and dissonance, especially if these relate to the sacred core of the hospital order, its welfare orientation and medical science frame.

172. Discourses are cultural artefacts, formulated according to certain rules – in a given institutional context – about the form, property context. Thus, the utterances, arguments, statements, making up a discourse (Ellingson, 1995) assume or refer to particular definitions of the situation, within a specific normative-cognitive frame.

There are correct and incorrect ways of formulating sentences, statements, or discourses – which have not been determined by the individual – even powerful agents are constrained in this respect.

173. In 1968, the Ad Hoc Committee of the Harvard Medical School declared that individuals in an irreversible coma who were diagnosed as having "braindead syndrome" could be declared dead. The procedure to determine death entailed identifying the following signs: (a) absence of cerebral responsiveness; (b) absence of induced or spontaneous movements; (c) absence of spontaneous respiration (requiring respirator); (d) absence of cephalic and deep-tendon reflexes; (e) absence of drug intoxication or hypothermia; (f) presence of a flat EEG; (g) persistence of these conditions for 24 hours. This procedure is not universally valid, its basic tenets varying in different states and countries. But this protocol and variants of it serve to define reality, to legitimise particular judgements and actions – and the cognitions grounded in or associated with these – and to define contrary cognitions as illegitimate or irrelevant. The Pittsburgh Protocol refers to a procedure initiated in several US hospitals to make use of non-heart beating donors (NHBD) (see Chapter 10, note on NHBD).

174. Other types of strategy in stabilising the cognitions of people with whom one is dealing – who might act or express themselves in ways which would cause organisational dissonance – are typically concealment and public image-making. Reports on non-public discourses and procedures are common (and are also observable in the settings we have studied). For instance, the unwritten rule of not talking about "inappropriate" feelings is relaxed enough sometimes to permit discussion, but the privacy that surrounds these infrequent occasions suggests the degree to which the taboo exists (Smith and Kleinman, 1989); or in the situations described by Youngner (1990): "Practising intubation and other techniques on cadavers is widespread, but done largely in secret and without the permission of families. It remains a controversial and potential rancorous issue...The parallels with organ retrieval for transplantation seem clear; if anything, its unique circumstance serve to heighten our society's ambivalence". Similar is the description of organ extraction from a non-heart-beating-donor in DeVita et al. (1993:377): "All health team members agreed that it would have been very difficult and stressful to have had the family present in the OR (operation room) at any time during the process because (1) the OR is an unfamiliar, cold and antiseptic environment for the family; (2) the short time between death pronouncement and organ procurement would not have allowed the family sufficient time to grieve; (3) the juxtaposition of the transplant team in the next room and the family in the OR with the patient would have been uncomfortable for at least some members of the team". Lack of space prevents us from exploring these aspects of cognitive stabilisation further.

175. In the case of a non-medical profession dealing directly with clients, Blau (1955) also notes the professionals' common use of derogatory names, standardised complaints and jokes about their clients as a way to cope with the tensions and conflicts arising in

their dealings with their clients (Blau, 1955). Such communicative actions, he argues, serve to differentiate the professionals from the clients and to reinforce their own solidarity. At the same time, they maintain an image of themselves vis-à-vis clients as capable and concerned professionals rationally dealing with client problems, thus ignoring, re-defining, transforming contradictory messages, events, data.

Jokes about clients among professionals serve to reduce the experience of dissonance and distress from challenges and complaints. Blau (1955: 91-92) observes: "The integrative experience of common amusement was based on common disidentification with ridiculous clients. Stupid, hostile, impertinent, or mentally deranged applicants, although admittedly exceptional, were often responsible for conflicts and lent themselves particularly well to being ridiculed. Funny tales were preoccupied with these clients, producing a stereotype with which the interviewer could hardly sympathise." Moreover, the laughing social approval of inconsiderate treatment of these clients created or reinforced group norms. Jokes not only reduced or dissolved dissonant experiences, self-reproach, and uncertainty that had risen in the past but also forestalled their occurrence in future cases of a similar kind. They transformed acts of inconsiderate treatment of clients from a private exception into a socially approved practice. Of course, this worked to the detriment of many agencies' clients. "Ridicule of clients is, of course, an expression of aggression against them. The interviewer's jokes, however, just like his complaints, also served to absolve him from guilt feelings ... laughter is the social evidence of the stupidity of clients – and not of any mistake of the professionals..." (Blau, 1955:91-92).

As discourses, jokes differ from complaints. The latter are listened to as an expression of solidarity with the speaker and sympathy with his difficulties. They therefore presupposed social cohesion, whereas jokes were instrumental in creating or increasing solidarity by uniting a group in the pleasant experience of laughter together. Jokes were often told to a group while complaints were nearly always made to a single colleague. Since jokes were intended to deal with generic client types, most members of the audience could remember some of their own clients who "do things like that". Latent doubts and guilt feelings of listeners as well as those of the speaker were dispelled by the common laughter at such "crazy" clients (Blau, 1955: 92).

176. Note that this theory suggests an alternative to organisational design and development based on assumptions of rationality.

177. Within the medical profession there is a powerful ideology of affective neutrality – and the orientation of "detached concern" in dealing with patients (Fox, 1988; 1989:85-87). Affective neutrality refers to the ability of an actor to inhibit inappropriate feelings such as repulsion, anger, sexual arousal etc. towards patients; or to control or transform feelings that one violates the sanctity of the body when operating on or dealing with corpses etc. The capacity for detachment and emotional neutrality is part and parcel of "professionalisation". Medical students acquire in part this orientation during their studies, as a process of cognitive re-framing where they

learn to conceptually and discursively separate body from person. In the settings which we have investigated this means a conceptualisation (and related discourses) transforming the personalised deceased into a "corpse".

Detachment then seems to be a result of disciplination, a learned professional response to uncomfortable feelings aroused in transgressing social taboos associated with having contact with people (i.e. their bodies), not just an individual response but a socially structured one. Accordingly, many of the previously cited experiences towards the braindead are reported not to be the same for all the medical staff. Physicians appear to have more "distance", or greater affective neutrality, towards cadavers than nurses who are trained differently and occupy different positions in the hospital system (Sanner:1991:210), even if professional detachment is present in the case of nurses also. As one nurse puts it (also, see Fox, 1990), nurses do not necessarily lack feeling and compassion; they are distancing themselves, trying not to feel strongly. Otherwise, they cannot function as well in such stressful situations.

Inappropriate, "unprofessional" feelings are learned, to a greater or lesser extent, to be effectively suppressed during medical training, even if no specific techniques to achieve this are taught to the students (Smith and Kleinman, 1989). Despite anticipatory socialisation, many medical students experience considerable discomfort in connection with anatomy and autopsy training (Fox, 1989:86). These feelings are based on the fact that the dead bodies with which they have contact were people; the students feel uncertain about the relationship of the person to the body, a relationship they had previously taken for granted (Smith and Kleinman, 1989). In addition, studies on medical culture suggest that autopsies are more upsetting to medical students than dissection because the body is "freshly dead"; it still retains some personhood (name, personal history in the form of the patient's medical record). There are obviously grades of life and death, and confrontation with death as "recent life" is apparently much more disconcerting than dealing with the cadavers in the anatomy laboratory (Fox, 1989:86). One medical student put it graphically when explaining that the freshly dead body is "much closer to life than the smoked herring (cadaver) in gross anatomy" (Smith and Kleinman (1989:58)).

In spite of an ethos of professional detachment and procedures to concentrate on a single body part or zone, dealing with dead persons as if they are alive clashes with other aspects of health care professionalism, namely to help patients that one deals with. Gentleman et al. (1990:1205) reports: "Some of the patients who die without ever being ventilated are admitted to hospital soon after an acute brain insult, commonly a head injury or intracranial haemorrhage. Others suffer an acute incident when already in the hospital, such as a cardiac arrest or a recurrent subarachnoid haemorrhage or some other sudden relapse or deterioration. When it is evident that the prognosis is hopeless a decision is made not to start ventilation because it would be futile. Some anaesthetists and nurses are not prepared to ventilate such patients with the specific intention of providing donor organs, and this was the reaction of staff in our unit during recent discussions. One objection is reluctance to embark on a major intervention with no prospect of helping the patient, another is unwillingness to commit professional time and other intensive care resources in these circumstances."

178. This reduces, of course, the surgeon's awareness of the patient as a whole person, while the surgeon is engaged in cutting into, "wounding", removing or implanting, and sewing up a human being; but draping the patient is not just an aseptic technique but also has an important relationship to respecting the dignity of the anaesthetised patient (Fox, 1989: 579).

179. This is not to claim that the techniques and technologies serve only ritualistic purposes, that they are neither instrumental nor effective in many instances for making judgements. Rather, the emphasis here is simply on their social and cognitive functions. Many of the problems identified here relate to Mary Douglas' characterisation of problem situations where there is a lack of clear boundaries (that is, there is ambiguity related to a matter that is sacred or highly value-laden) between significant categories. Many rituals (and ceremonies) reaffirm the sacredness of collective selves, their representatives, their core values, and normative order including authority and status relations. There is no contradiction between a commitment to the interaction ritual and the collective selves, and commitment to key institutionalised values or role performance. They make up a field.

180. Theories of ritual can be divided into two schools (Bell, 1992). One school stresses the distinctiveness of ritual, contrasting the ritual/magical activity as rule governed – routinised – symbolic or non instrumental activity with the technical/utilitarian activity as pragmatic and instrumentally effective. However, in my view, the distinction between symbolic and utilitarian aspects is a matter of degree. Ritual as a cathartic anxiety reducer can be regarded as both. Above all, however, ritual is a form of communication composed of culturally normalised acts that have become distinctive by being diverted to special functions where they are given magical efficacy; it is an effective means of socially regulating actors' orientations, definitions of the situation, experiences (Bell, 1992:178, 183-186).

181. Ritual action is ostensibly behavioural, physical, whereas discourse is more clearly talk. But there is not clear boundary, since much ritual entails talking and verbal communication and a discourse may be read or presented in highly ritualistic ways with gestures and bodily movements.

182. This relates to Giddens' (1984) important observation that people adhere to routines in their interaction in order to avoid anxiety.

183. Members of any group or collectivity may experience daily tensions and conflicts that contradict norms of solidarity and the vision of peaceful life together. They engage in rituals and ceremonies which redefine the reality. Many daily experiences are redefined as not "reality". Reality becomes that defined by the ritual, the other experience is ephemeral.

184. Of course, this is surely related to the association Turner (1969) and Malinowski (1951) saw between rituals and social crises – in part to minimise the impact of crises. Malinowski (1951) saw also such a connection between ritual and crises or profound

changes/passages such as illness, birth, marriage, death, transition and socialisation to new roles and statuses (see Wolf, 1988).

185. While the form of giving and taking orders is the ceremonial core of any work organisation – the superordinate acting authoritatively and expecting compliance and subordinates showing deference and appearing to act dutifully – Collins (1988:205) stresses that in practice, managers and directors are less than fully effective in controlling those under them. The superordinates know this in many instances, but they go through the ritual nevertheless as a theatrical performance, in which both sides know and perform their parts.

186. Ritual communicates a great deal that would be difficult to express in words, in part because of ambiguity and irony in the message. As Bosk observes (1979:144): "...putting on the hair shirt ...emphasises the surgeon's charity, humanity, and the scope of his wisdom ...It allows him to express guilt without being consumed by it...At the same time, it communicates to subordinates that no one is perfect; it models for them the proper expression of guilt and teaches them to accept that such accidents are an inevitable, unfortunate, and intractable part of professional life."

187. The constitution, regulation, and stabilisation of the medical order depends on a stable/stabilised cognitive-normative frame. It also depends on concrete social processes, sanctions, rituals, and discourses, that stabilise collective representations, classification schemes, key cognitions, judgements, and commitments.

188. There is, however, a scientific controversy internal to the profession about where to establish lower brain stem or higher as the decisive criteria and about the accuracy of "brain death" certification.

189. The orders of some organisations are based largely on coercion and physical constraint (e.g. prisons and closed mental hospitals) or on remuneration (people do what they do and obey authority in exchange for wages or salaries). But even these depend on some mutual trust and interdependence among those exercising power, applying or threatening to apply coercive measures or remunerative measures.

190. Nurses are educated in the medical science perspective, although not with the same intensity and determination as physicians. This perspective does not always suit or function comfortably with the "nursing and care" orientation of nurses. Considerations of this issue would take us beyond the scope of this chapter.

191. Of course, an organisation may be "too open", ready to adjust and adapt their cognitions and cognitive frame to all incoming signals and data, no matter how inconsistent, irrelevant, etc. thereby eliminating the sense of cognitive or social stability. As a result, there is no collective order. One might conclude that the ideal is a balance between adaptability/adjustment and internal order and stability. But this is precisely one of the major challenges to organisational leadership (whether concentrated or diffused, organically throughout the organisation).

192. The bureaucratic type of organisation (and hospitals belong to this category), is the model of the rational organisation. However, vague or ambiguous task assignments are submitted at the top respective bottom of the hierarchical pyramidal form of the

bureaucratic organisation.

193. The Board of Health includes in the category of "minor incisions" (or "small parts"): the bone tissue that surrounds hipbone and knee prosthesis, biological material from the bladder, penis, heart valve to the aorta, and a thin slice of muscle from the leg and arm. But also includes from half to one square centimeter of liver tissue, vesicula biliar, pancreas, stomach, duodenum, small intestine, colon, aorta, bladder and ovary, fragments of arteries and veins, and of muscle. Pieces of tissue of a maximum of one square centimeter of the musculus soleus, tiroidal tissue, pieces of "earbones", and of front teeth. However, incisions as the following are not considered minor according to the Board: one centimeter pieces of arteries from the hands, two grams of prostate tissue, three centimeter segments of the "large arteries", pieces of brain tissue of about ten grams, one square decimeter of undamaged lung tissue, 5x5 cm pieces of veins from hands, the eye or the hypophysis (SOU 1989:98:197).

194. The dead body occupies a legally undefined place as the physical enactment of the actor's rational intentions. The increasing use of body organs/tissue in medical therapy sanctions a view of human body parts as useful "matter", at the same time that dead persons are to be treated with "piety". The sacredness of the dead body is officially underscored. The gap in the denotation of bodies/organs for transplantation, in the patient-centred medical practice and the citizen-centred discourse of the legal tradition, entails tensions.

195. One aspect of rationality is equivalent to self-disciplination, self-control (opposite to uncontrolled behaviour). In everyday practice more than just young children and mentally disabled are downgraded: partially or non-acculturated foreign nationals (inappropriate behaviour) or the "self-abusers" such as, drug addicts, alcoholics, smokers (lack of control), and why not including at least to a certain extent the chronically unemployed and less educated (poorly disciplined, and badly articulated (verbal or written articulation is an important measure of rational aptitude)). This idea can be summarised as: low self-disciplination equal to low rationality equal to low legal agency.

196. Boundaries and meanings vary depending on situational contexts, and these are social and cultural ones. A "body" can be, for example, conceived as material, physiological, aesthetic, sexual or moral entity, this depending on the perspective applied.

197. Which conception is to be applied is not commonly a question of individual choice but collective definitions (often as a result of power struggles) and authority.

198. The rights of individuals have increased historically (Inger, 1985) and this historical process can be understood as a development towards the realisation of the civil ideal of citizen rights and liberties. The right ascribed to an individual in more traditional societies was related to the person's family and community roles but the modern state has become a major collective source of individual identity defined as citizenship, that confers rights on citizens, but also establishes its jurisdiction and regulations.

199. The Council of Law (*lågradet*) is appointed to oversee that new laws are not opposed to the constitution. The courts are dispensed from applying a law that contradicts

constitutional law.

200. In many cases injuries during medical procedures or medical actions with proper consent does not seem to entail serious (civil or criminal) legal consequences for medical and nursing personnel.

201. The category of full capable adult citizen is synonymous with the Person, and thus constitutes the axial and tacit category. The other categories (for example minor or mentally incompetent) are – from the perspective of rights over body – reduced variants, that is with lesser degree of attributions.

202. In this simple model (and hereafter) I treat "the state" as a single level, when in fact there are three distinct levels in Sweden: central or proper state, county and municipality levels. Laws such as the body of laws discussed in this chapter are legislated at the central level as parliamentary acts. The National Board of Health and Welfare (Socialstyrelsen) provides more detailed guidelines regarding the application of the laws. The use of bodies and organ parts has to follow the national legislation, but operationally lower units such as hospital units are typically in direct control.

203. That is the degree of invasiveness of the procedure, its later consequences (irreversibility, etc.).

204. Two medical actions take the age of the individual into consideration, sterilisation and castration (including change of sex). Persons under 25 years old (for sterilization) and 23 years old (for castration) need special authorization in order to obtain these procedures. This may be related to the irreversibility of the procedure.

205. Cultural values in the legal system can also be found in the sphere of the application of the laws, that is the courts, but this appears to be less relevant in Sweden than for common law systems. The courts have to take into consideration international conventions, general policies (e.g. United Nations Declaration of Human Rights), and additionally non-juridical factors are present in the judicial sphere such as established moral rights (e.g. parent's right to bestow care upon her own children). However, the study of cultural values in the exercise of the law is beyond the scope of this chapter.

206. However, two important exceptions are indicated, where societal rights take total prevalence over individual rights in medical procedures regarding living persons. A patient is compelled to submit to treatment or preventive measures in the case of dangerous contagious diseases and also in the treatment of psychic illnesses under specifically defined conditions. Regarding deceased persons, autopsies and body tissue extraction are performed without any consent.

207. General consent is an unspecified form of consent, e.g. silent consent, presumed consent or hypothetical consent.

208. Soldiers (under service) are an exception in this regard.

209. A legal tutor acts as next-of-kin in the case of minors and mentally disabled.

210. General medical instruction, 10§ p1.

211. Government's Propostion 1978/79:220 pp. 20 and 45.

212. However, if a minor clearly refuses that information regarding medical procedures will be given to the parents or adults in charge, this should be respected (and special support

should be given to the woman before and after the abortion) (Sjolenius, 1991).

213. The physician evaluates the situation from case to case (Sjolenius, 1989) but is generally accepted that around puberty or 15 years old a person is capable of deciding about most treatments.

214. Object of right: object of a legal right, cannot have rights or duties.

215. In the middle ages, in retaliation for an offence, whole kin or entire villages were punished.

216. The requirements of information and consultation are to a certain extent relative (Act on Supervision to Health Care Personnel 1980:11 5§).

217. Pollock and Maitland give historical examples of partial actors, "self-unable" (or near so) to take action before the law and who depended on a legally capable social actor that actuated as "the acting self". Examples of these were the guardian in the case of minors and disabled; the husband that acted as the agent of the wife (or the father if the woman was unmarried); the church was the agent of monks and the nuns (who had renounced to their civil rights). Common to semi-actors such as minors, women, handicapped etc. was the lack of status of full personhood in the public sphere.

218. Some authors place women as part of this group of socially dis-abled as persons with partial personhood. Women's rights over the body can conflict with what is defined as "the rights of mature foetuses in the womb" (these endowed with rights as potential persons). In this case the foetus as another partial actor has the state as a trustee.

219. The intentionality of the physician in doing what according to her is the best for the patient appears to be a common rationale behind the leniency in disciplinary measures, but also reflects the legal unclarity about patient's rights regarding services provided by state hospitals (Rynning, 1994).

220. However, a guideline from the National Board of Health (SoS) regarding the LVM (Act on the Care of Abusers, 1983:3 4) states: "The risk for the foetus – if a woman cannot abstain from her abuse of alcohol and/or narcotics – has to be understood as a sign that the woman has lost control over her abuse, and that she should receive care for her abuse. The rationale is the endangerment of the woman's psychological health if she becomes responsible for a child born with serious damages (Socialutskottet 1981,6). Notwithstanding, according to the Secrecy Act, an authority (e.g. a psychiatric institution or social assistant) cannot give information about the particular situation of the woman to a Maternity Care Centre.

221. Emergency (nödvärn) is regulated in BrB 24:4, and its application has to be justified by safeguarding among other things "life and health" (both the patient's and other individuals' life and health). However, to attempt suicide is not forbidden by law, and the (surviving) person does not have to follow any medical treatment after the attempt (Sjölenius, 84-85).

222. The attitude of the patient is the defining factor in the application of the LTP (Act on Forensic Psychiatric Care), that is the patient clearly refuses medical treatment, or shows evident signs of lacking mental capacity to express her will about the treatment.

223. Mechanical actions on bodies seem to be more regulated than the use of, e.g.,

neuroleptics. For example, to give electroshock to a patient without her consent must be exceptional; mechanical restraints should not be applied for more than a few hours and the patient should be under surveillance; and no patient may be kept isolated more that 8 hours.

224. An important societal value or good may be the protection of women's rights, e.g. the right to have an abortion or to be free of the threat of violence from men or their husbands. Societies assign value to life, for example the life of a developed foetus. This value is weighed against the value of protecting women's rights in the case of, for instance, abortion. Hence the rule in Sweden, where concern for the foetus enters into the regulation, and the Socialstyrelsen is empowered to make a determination on a case-by-case basis. Theoretically, the Socialstyrelsen could decide in favour of the foetus, denying the right of abortion to the mother. They could also decide in favour of the mother and against the foetus.

225. According to Foucault, disciplinary technicians, for example, teachers, psychologists, psychiatrists or social workers, act as normative judges, differentiating, quantifying and ranking individuals according to their abilities to conform to the normative indications of each disciplinary technology.

226. Organ transplantation not only creates problems in the relationship of medical personnel with next-of-kin, but also for those professionals who must try to persuade and deal with the next-of-kin of deceased and also to deal with dead bodies. Typically, there are two distinct ways of facing these problems: (1) objectification – a dead person is a corpse, she has no personality; and is separated from her soul and her network of people; and (2) subjectification – a dead person enjoys sacrality, belongs to a network of living people, and cannot be treated as lacking in personality and soul. The world of sacrality and soul can be engaged. But not with technical and "rational" means. But only through special rituals and ceremonies that acknowledge that something valuable, even sacred is "donated", and that this is a part of community solidarity, and certainly not an administrative or technical or other instrumental activity.

227. The recipients of living donor kidneys tend to be younger and belong to a good-risk category, with a better psychosocial environment, that could also contribute to a better compliance and higher survival rate (McMaster and Czerniak (1991:37)).

228. While most Western legislations protect individual right to (bodily) integrity, the adult individual is entitled to voluntarily abstain from these constitutional rights and give (informed) consent to the extraction of one paired organ for purposes of transplantation. However, given the unclarity about the superior benefits in living organ donation, the main argumentation lines favouring the practice, are clearly pragmatic (see Jakobsen et al., 1991; Bonomini, 1991).

229. Important studies about consent in medical procedures, particularly for surgical patients, has shown that informed consent is practically non-existent (Lisz and Meisel (1982)). For example, Rynning (1994) points out that, in Sweden, many medical interventions are taken without proper consent in the legal sense, and that this infringement can take place without any legal sanction, or with minimum disciplinary sanctions under the

implicit assumption of "good intent and expertise".

230. To this contributes the hierarchical structure of the hospital (a professional bureaucracy) with the physician at the top, an unfamiliar place for most lay people and where you go only when you are sick and need help (with the exception of women).

231. There is no sociological task to pronounce verdicts about what "should be done" in this matter. However, the stringency of a strict market regulation (formal regulation) would fit badly with this type of transaction. Likewise the control of the state administration in warranting compliance to those eventual market rules would create an enormous bureaucratic structure. Network organisations or clans (Ouchi (1991)) are arguably the best forms of regulating social transactions when the nature of the item transferred is unclear (organ donation can also be understood as mainly a transfer of services).

232. Another ethically problematic issue concerns the use of non-heart beating donors (NHBD). This type of donor is defined as a non-braindead donor (the braindead donor is the common case) whose heart or circulatory system has ceased to function. Organ donation from NHBDs was initiated a few years ago in several US hospitals. An example of NHBD is the following: the patient is terminally ill or suffers a serious neurological damage and is not expected to ever regain consciousness. The family decides that life support should be withdrawn, and that afterwards her organs may be donated. From this moment on the patient receives "comfort measures only" and is taken to the operation theatre. Here the patient is sedated and the life support is withdrawn. After several minutes without vital signs, the patient is pronounced dead. The organs are removed immediately thereafter (De Vita et al., 1993b). The use of NHBDs is highly controversial. It is, on the one hand, defended and ethically justified by the endemic organ shortage, on the other hand, the procedure appears to be questionable since death can be certified after two minutes of ceasing of circulatory and respiratory functions; it can hasten death, does not provide good care for dying patients or for their families (Spielman and Simmons, 1995); and risks defiling the life-saving character of the OP with a disquieting effect on the surgical team (Fox, 1993).

233. The latest proposed alternative to solve the problem of organ shortage is to use animal organs – eventually genetically engineered in order to make them more akin to human tissue and more easily accepted by the recipient. Apart from the epidemiological risks of activating animal retrovirus in the human receiver (with unknown consequences), the ethical issue at stake would appear to be the lack of moral justification in utilising animals – since they can neither be regarded as donors nor can they understand the motive behind their sacrifice. The ecological-philosophical arguments used against this practice are based on the logical impossibility of proving that (a) humans and animals are endowed with a radically different nature, (b) that even if a radical difference could be established, it would hardly justify killing them for the purpose of expropriating their organs for the benefit of human populations. In any case, several xenotransplantations have been already performed and even if no patient has survived the implantation more than a few days, experiments are being conducted at present in a strictly controlled form.

234. In my view, we already have indications of this normalisation process in the lack of

articulation of whatever reservations or doubts people can have, and moreover when people do express reservations about donation, these are often referred to as a result of some personal inadequacy. This is not surprising, since the attitudes of non-positive groups, sometimes called "free riders" or "uneducated public" has been explained as lack of adequate information in the mildest variants, to psychological instability and lower IQ in the more bizarre ones.

235. In a not too distant European past, the bodies of the "unworthy" could be freely expropriated, and this type of action not only reopens old wounds but is deeply incompatible with modern democracy.

236. A widely recognised phenomena in organ donation is the reluctance of the physicians to retrieve an organ if the relatives of the deceased are opposed to it, independently of what is stated in the legislation. The ethical principle of voluntarism in organ donation is apparently not consistent with the role of relatives vetoing an individual organ donation (Land et al., 1991). Arguments favouring the donation in spite of family opposition pivot on the importance of legal and moral rectitude, medical responsibility towards waiting patients. It is noteworthy in that opposition to autopsies are uncommon (though a similar mutilation of the corpse takes place).

237. For example, in the Swedish legislation the introduction of presumed consent has been legitimised by the fact that a majority of the Swedes were positive towards organ donation (Sanner, 1993, 1994; Gäbel and Lindskoug, 1989; Gäbel et al., 1992). To rely on the opinion of majorities is a fine democratic tradition, but what is the percent that establishes the line between the ethical or non-ethical in presumed consent, 51%, 66% of the population? How are non-respondents to be categorised? Added arguments were the need of organs for transplantation [a practical notion] and the reduced costs of kidney transplants when compared to dialysis [notion of effectivity].

238. By 1968, the Ad Hoc Committee of the Harvard Medical School declared that individuals with irreversible coma who were to be diagnosed as having "brain death syndrome" could be declared dead. Its signs were defined as: (a) absence of cerebral responsiveness, (b) absence of induced or spontaneous movements, (c) absence of spontaneous respiration (requiring respirator), (d) absence of cephalic and deep-tendon reflexes, (e) absence of drug intoxication or hypothermia, (f) presence of a flat EEG, (g) persistence of these conditions for 24 hours. This legal model is far from universally valid since its definition varies somewhat in different countries. Brain death is commonly defined as the complete and irreversible loss of all brain functions (while intensive care and mechanical respiration initially keep the remaining parts of the body alive).

239. The supply-demand gap can be reduced also by encouraging donation or changing criteria for donation (through legal or medical redefinitions). It also can be indirectly reduced by avoiding wastage through an effective communication net.

240. Each institutional domain is based on particular types of social relationships or social rule systems, each with its own distinct logic or rationality (Burns and Flam, 1987:75; Burns and Dietz, 1996). Each rationality involves not only specific organising principles and transaction rules, but a jurisdiction of meaning. It defines and distinguishes the

legitimate actors (to be included, respectively excluded) in the collective activity, the proper types of actions and interactions to be performed in the particular setting, the appropriate or proper places and times to engage in the activity.

241. Not all moral claims throughout an OTS have the same legitimacy and level of articulation, but given the characteristic of the organisation – where the organ procurement depends on people's willingness to donate – public values and beliefs weigh more than they otherwise would in the professional bureaucracy of the hospital.

242. However, Schluchter (1981) adds a third ethical position to Weber's classification that he baptises "ethics of adjustment", where morality is subordinated to efficiency. An ethics of adjustment – for example, the pragmatism of the market – is problematic in that it leads to the violation and erosion of important social values and ethical principles, not just in general or vague terms, but risks eroding the same values that ultimately support the market itself, that is respect for agreed terms of the transactions, not cheating, etc. (Burns, 1995). This is also a risk in the area of modern medicine where, as Fox stresses in a number of her works, there are tendencies toward a powerful pragmatism at the expense of morality.

243. The demand for bodies, organs and tissue in medical research is considerable, but also in medical education (anatomy), in the preparation of therapeutic extracts, and particularly in transplantation. The usefulness of bodies and body parts has propelled most states to introduce legal changes in death criteria and laws concerning removal and use of organs.

Bibliography

References: Swedish Governmental Documents

Swedish Legislative Propositions

Proposition 1978/79:220 (Governmental) om samhällets tillsyn över hälso-och sjukvårdspersonalen m.fl.

Proposition 1994/95:148 (Governmental) Transplantationer och obduktioner m.m.

Swedish Government Official Reports (SOU)

SOU 1936/46 *Betänkande angående sterilisering.* Swedish Government Official Report. Stockholm.

SOU 1974:25 *Fri Sterilisering.* Betänkande av Steriliseringsutredningen.

SOU 1989:98 *Transplantation. Etiska, medicinska och rättsliga aspekter.* Betänkande av transplantationsutredningen.

SOU 1989:99 *Organdonation och transplantation. Psykologiska aspekter. Samtal med vårdpersonal, anhöriga och allmänheten.* M. Sanner. Rapport utgiven av transplantationsutredningen.

SOU 1992:16 *Kroppen efter döden.* Slutbetänkande av transplantationsutredningen.

Reports by the Swedish Board of Health

SoS 1988:19. Socialstyrelsen redovisar.*Transplantationsverksamhet för Lever och Hjärta.*

General References

Abelson, R., E. Aronson, W. McGuire, T. Newcomb, M. Rosenberg and P. Tannenbaum (eds) (1968) *Theories of Cognitive Consistency: A Sourcebook.* Chicago: Rand McNally.

Abuna, G., M. Sabawi, M. Kumar and M. Samham (1991) "The Negative Aspect of Paid Donation" in Land, W. and J.B. Dossetor.

ACCORD. Australian Coordinating Committee on Organ Registries and Donation (1995) "Organ donation attitudes research" (performed by Frank Small and Associates).

Acquili, E., C. Laughlin and J. McManus (1979) *The Spectrum of Ritual*. New York: Columbia University Press.

Alföldy, F. (1997) The History of Transplantation http://transito.sote.hu/hist.htm.

Alter, C. and J. Hage (1993) *Organizations Working Together*. Newbury Park: Sage.

Anbäcken, O. (1985) *Patientmedverkan och organisationsstruktur: En studie om patientens roll och funktion i vårdorganisationen* (Patient Involvement and Organization Structure). Linköping: Linköping Studies in Management and Economics.

Andersson Wretmark, A. (1994) "Ritual och ritual för dödfödda och tidigt döda barn". *Socialmedicinsk Tidskrift*. Nr.7-8, pp. 310-314.

Anspach, R. (1993) *Deciding Who Lives. Fateful Choices in the Intensive Care Nursery*. University of California Press.

ANZOD *Registry Report* (1997) Australia and New Zealand Organ Donation Registry, Adelaide, South Australia. Editors: K. Herbertt, G.R. Russ.

Arnold, R. and S. Youngner (1993) "The Dead Donor Rule: Should We Stretch It, Bend It, Abandon It?". *Kennedy Institute of Ethics Journal*. Vol. 3 (No. 2): 263-278.

Aronson, E. (1968) "Dissonance Theory: Progress and Problems" in R. P. Abelson, E. Aronson, W.J. McGuire, T. M. Newcomb, M.J. Rosenberg and P. H. Tannenbaum (eds).

Aronson, E. (1969) "The Theory of Cognitive Dissonance: A Current Perspective" in L. Berkowitz (ed.) *Advances in Experimental Social Psychology*, Vol. 4. New York: Academic Press (pp. 1-34).

Aronson, E. (1995) *The Social Animal* (7th edition). New York: W.H. Freeman.

Aronson, E. and J.M.Carlsmith (1963) "Effect of the Severity of Threat on the Devaluation of Forbidden Behavior". *Journal of Abnormal and Social Psychology*, Vol. 66:584-588.

Aronson, E. and J.Mills (1959) "The Effect of Severity of Initiation on Liking for a Group". *Journal of Abnormal and Social Psychology*, Vol. 59:177-181.

Arrow, K. (1981) Chapter in Marshall Cohen, T. Nagel and T. Scanlon (eds) *Medicine and Moral Philosophy*. Princeton, New Jersey: Princeton University Press.

Atkins, K. (1992) "The Body and the Person in Organ Transplants". *The Australian Nurses Journal* (July) Vol. 22 (No. 1).

Bailey, J. (1989) "Female drinking drivers in New Zealand" in M. Valverius (ed.) *Women, Alcohol, Drugs and Traffic.* Proceedings of the International Workshop, September 29-30, 1989.

Banta, D., I. Karlberg and T. Schersten (1989) "Organtransplantationer. Samband mellan volym, resultat och kostnad -en litteratur översikt". *Statens Beredning för Utvärdering av medicinsk metodik (SBU).* December. Stockholm.

Barnard, C.I. (1938) *The functions of the Executive.* Cambridge: Harvard University Press.

Baumgartner, T. and T.R.Burns (1984) *Transitions to Alternative Energy Systems: Entrepreneurs, New Technologies and Social Change.* Boulder, Colorado/London: Westview Press.

Beirness, D. (1989) "Female Drivers in Canada: Trends in Accident Involvement" in M. Valverius (ed.) *Women, Alcohol, Drugs and Traffic.* Proceedings of the International Workshop, September 29-30, 1989.

Bell, C. (1992) *Ritual Theory, Ritual Practice.* New York: Oxford University Press.

Bergström, C., L. Svensson, A. Wolfbrandt and M. Lundell (on behalf of the Swedish Transplant Coordinators) (1997) "The Swedish Transplant Coordinators Experience of the New Transplantation Act and the Donor Register 1Year After Implementation". *Transplantation Proceedings* 29, 3232-3233.

Bidwell, C.E. (1976) "The Structure of Professional Help" in Loubser, J. et al. (eds) *Explorations in General Theory in Social Science: Essays in Honor of Talcott Parsons.* New York: Free Press.

Billig, M. (1982) *Ideology and Social Psychology.* Oxford: Basil Blackwell.

Billig, M., S. Condor, D. Edwards, M. Gain, D. Middleton and A. Radley (1988) *Ideological Dilemmas.* London: Sage.

Blau, P. (1956) *The Dynamics of Bureaucracy: A Study of Interpersonal Relations in Two Government Agencies.* Chicago: University of Chicago Press.

Blau, P. and W.R. Scott (1962) *Formal Organizations: A Comparative Approach.* San Francisco: Chandler.

Blohmé, I., I. Fehrman and G. Nordén (1992) "Living Donor Nephrectomy. Complicating Rates in 490 Consecutive Cases". *Scandinavian Journal of Urology and Nephrology,* 26:149-153.

Bos, M. and J. Wilmink (1991) "Attitudes to Using Living Related Kidney Donors in the Netherlands" in Land, W. and J.B. Dossetor (eds) *Organ Replacement Therapy: Ethics, Justice, Commerce.* First Joint Meeting of ESOT and EDTA/ERA. Munich. December. Springer Verlag.

Bosk, C.L. (1979) *Forgive and Remember: Managing Medical Failure.* Chicago: The University of Chicago Press.

Bosk, C.L. (1980) "Occupational Rituals in Patient Management". *New England Journal of Medicine,* Vol. 303, No. 2: 71-76.

Bourdieu, P. (1991) *Language and Symbolic Power.* Cambridge: Harvard University Press.

Bradach, J.L. and R. G. Eccles (1989) "Price, authority and trust: from ideal types to plural forms". *Annual Review of Sociology,* 15:97-118.

Brante, T. and M. Hallberg (1989) "Kontroversen om dodsbegreppet", *Vest.*

Braun, I. (1994) "Winged Dinosaurs: On Intersystem Network of Large Technical Systems", manuscript.

Braun, I. and B. Joerges (1993) "How to Recombine Large Systems: the Case of European Organ Transplantation", *Report   FSII   93-905.* Wissenschaftszcentrum: Berlin.

Brehm, J. and A. Cohen (1962) *Explorations in Cognitive Dissonance.* New York: Wiley.

Briggs, J.D., A. Crombie, J. Fabre, E. Major, J. Thorogood and P.S. Veitch (1997) "Dialysis and transplantation news. Organ donation in the UK: a survey by a British Transplantation Society working party". *Nephrology Dialysis and Transplantation,* Vol. 12, 11: November.

Broberg, G. and M. Tydén (1991) *Oönskade i Folkhemmet.* Gidlunds.

Brulle, R.J. (1994) "Power, Discourse and Social Problems: Social Problems from a Rhetorical Perspective", in *Current Perspectives in Social Problems.* Vol. 5. Greenwich, Connecticut: JAI Press.

Bunzendahl, H., K. Wu, H. Kunsenbeck, G. Offner, U. Frei, H. Freyberger and R. Pichlmayr (1991) "Retrospective Evaluation of Psychosocial Factors in Former Living Related Kidney Donors" in Land, W. and J.B. Dossetor (eds) *Organ Replacement Therapy: Ethics, Justice, Commerce.* First Joint Meeting of ESOT and EDTA/ERA. Munich. December. Springer Verlag.

Burke, P. J. (1991) "Identity Processes and Social Stress", *American Sociological Review,* Vol. 56:836-849.

Burke, P. J. and D.C. Reitzes (1991) "An Identity Theory Approach to Commitment". *Social Psychology Quarterly,* Vol. 54:280-286.

Burns, T. and G. Stalker (1961) *The Management of Innovation.* London:

Tavistock Publications.

Burns, T.R. (1990) "Models of Social and Market Exchange: Toward a Sociological Theory of Games and Social Behavior" in C. Calhoun, M.W. Meyer and W.R. Scott (eds) *Structures of Power and Constraint: Papers in Honor of Peter M. Blau.* Cambridge: Cambridge University Press.

Burns, T.R. (1995) "Markets and Human Agency" in Carlo Mongardini (ed.) *L'Individuo e il mercato.* Rome: Bulzone Editore.

Burns, T.R., T. Baumgartner and P. De Ville (1985) *Man, decisions, society.* London/New York: Gordon & Breach.

Burns, T.R. and T. Dietz (1997) "Social Rule System Theory: Social Action, Institutional Arrangements and Evolutionary Processes" in R. Hollingsworth (ed.) *Social Actors and the Embeddedness of Institutions.* New York: M.E. Sharpe, 1995.

Burns, T.R. and E. Engdahl (1998) "The Social Construction of Mind: A socio-cultural perspective on language based consciousness". To appear in *Journal of Consciousness Studies*, Vol. 4, in press.

Burns, T.R. and H. Flam (1987) *The Shaping of Social Organization. Social Rule System Theory With Applications.* London: Sage 1987.

Burns, T.R., A. Gomolinska and D.Meeker in collaboration with P. DeVille and E. Griffor (1997) *The Dialectics of Social Action and Games: A General Mathematical Theory of Moral, Rational, and Creative Aspects of Knowing, Judging, and Interacting.* Uppsala. Uppsala Theory Circle Report, Department of Sociology.

Burns, T.R. and C. Laughlin (1979) "Ritual and the Resolution of Collective Action Problems" in Acquili, E., C. Laughlin and J. McManus (eds) *The Spectrum of Ritual.* New York: Columbia University Press.

Burns, T. R. and A. Midttun (1987) "Economic Growth, Environmentalism and Social Conflict: A Model of Hydro-power Planning in Norway", *Human System Management.*

Burns, T.R. and C. Sutton (1995) "Discourses, Institutions and Human Agency in Stability and Change". Paper presented at the Uppsala Theory Circle Workshop on "Discourse and Rhetoric: Social Science Perspectives". May 29-30, 1995, Uppsala, Sweden.

Burns, T.R. and R. Ueberhorst (1988) *Creative democracy: Systematic conflict resolution and policymaking in a world of high science and technology.* New York: Praeger.

Callender, C., J. Bayton and J. Clark (1982) "Attitudes Among Blacks Toward Donating Kidneys For Transplantation. A Pilot Project". *Journal of the National Medical Association*, pp. 807-809.

Chan, W. (1992) "The Role of the Operation Theatre in Organ Transplantation". *Transplantation Proceedings*, Vol. 24 (No. 5): 2042-2048.

Chapman, G. (1983) "Ritual and Rational Action in Hospitals". *Journal of Advanced Nursing*, 8: 13-20.

Cockerham, W. (1978) *Medical Sociology*. Englewood Cliffs, N.J.: Prentice-Hall.

Cohen, J. and A. Arato (1992) *Civil Society and Political Theory*. Cambridge: MIT Press.

Coleman, J.S. and E. Katz (1957) "The Diffusion of Innovation Among Physicians". *Sociometry*, Vol. 20 (No. 4).

Coleman, J.S., E. Katz and H. Menzel (1966) *Medical Innovation: A Diffusion Study*. Indianapolis: Bobbs-Merrill.

Collins, R. (1988) *Theoretical Sociology*. New York: Harcourt Jovanovich, Publishers.

Council of Europe (1997) ETS No.164 Convention for the protection of human rights and dignity of the human being with regard to the application of biology and medicine; Oviedo, 04.IV.1997.

Danish Council of Ethics (1989) "Death Criteria". *The Danish Council of Ethics first annual report*, 1988.

Davidson, M. and P. Devney (1991) "Attitudinal Barriers to Organ Donation Among Blacks". *Transplantation Proceedings*, pp.2531-2532.

Davis, F. (1989) "Organ Procurement and Transplantation". *Nursing Clinics of North America*, Vol. 2, No. 4 (December).

Davis, K. and E.E. Jones (1960) "Changes in Interpersonal Perception as a Means of Reducing Cognitive Dissonance". *Journal of Abnormal and Social Psychology*, Vol. 61:402-410.

De Vita, M. and J. Snyder (1993a) "Development of the University of Pittsburgh Medical Center Policy for the Care of Terminally Ill Patients Who May Become Organ Donors After Death Following the Removal of Life Support". *The Kennedy Institute of Ethics Journal*, Vol. 3 (No. 2): 131-143.

De Vita, M., Vukmir, R., Snyder, J. and Ch. Graziano (1993b) "Procuring Organs From A Non-Heart Beating Cadaver: A Case Report". *The Kennedy Institute of Ethics Journal*. Vol. 3 (No. 2):371-385.

Dennis, M. (1991) "How to think about making kidney transplantation equitable". Working paper 12. Local Justice Project. Department of Political Science. University of Chicago, Illinois.

Dennis, M., Herpin, N. and F. Peterson (1991) "The local justice of kidney transplantation in the US and France". Paper prepared for Local Justice Project in Poitiers, France, June.

DiMaggio, P. (1992) "Nadel's Paradox Revisited: Relational and Cultural Aspects of Organizational Structure", in Nohria and Eccles (eds).

Dominguez, J., F. Murillo Cabezas, A. Munoz Sanchez and M. Perez-San Gregorio (1992) "Psychological Aspects Leading to Refusal of Organ Donation in Southwest-Spain" in *Transplantation Proceedings*, Vol. 24 (No.1): 25-26.

Douglas, M. (1966) *Purity and Danger*. London: Routledge and Kegan Paul.

Douglas, M. (1986) *Risk Acceptability According to the Social Sciences*. London: Routledge and Kegan Paul.

Douglas, M. (1987) *How Institutions Think*. London: Routledge and Kegan Paul.

DuBose, E., R.Hamel and L. O'Conell (eds) (1994) *A Matter of Principles: Ferment in Bioethics*. Valley Forge, Penn: Trinity Press International.

Durkheim, E. (1976) *The Elementary Forms of the Religious Life*. London: George Allen & Unwin.

Eisenstein, Z. (1988) *The Female Body and the Law*. University of California Press.

Elias, N. (1996) *The Germans: Power Struggles and the Development of Habitus in the Nineteenth and Twentieth Centuries*. New York: Columbia University Press.

Elks, M.L. (1996) "Ritual and Roles in Medical Practice". *Perspectives in Biology and Medicine*, 39, 4, Summer, pp. 601-608.

Ellingson, S. (1995) "Understanding the Dialectic of Discourse and Collective Action: Public Debate and Rioting in Antebellum Cincinnati". *American Journal of Sociology*, Vol. 101: 101-44.

Emson, H.E. (1987) "The Ethics of Human Cadaver Organ Transplantation: A Biologist's Viewpoint". *Journal of Medical Ethics*, September 13(3): 124-126.

Etzioni, A. (1975) *Complex Organizations*. New York: Free Press.

Eurotransplant (1997) Version March 31, 1997.

Evans, R. (1992) "Need, demand and supply in organ transplantation". *Transplantation Proceedings*, Vol. 24 (No.5), pp. 2152-2154.

Expressen (1990) "Harriet fick sista remissen to London". Stockholm, January 6.

Faltin, D. (1992) "The decrease in organ donations from 1985 to 1990 caused by increasing medical contraindications and refusal by relatives". *Transplantation*, Vol. 54, 85-88, July.

Featherstone, M., M. Hepworth and B.S. Turner (1991) *The Body: Social Process and Cultural Theory*. London: Sage.

Fernandez Lucas, M., B. Miranda and R. Matesanz (1996) "Society and Professional Attitudes Towards Organ Donation" in Matesanz and Miranda.

Fernandez Lucas, M., E. Zayas, Z. Gonzalez, L. Morales Otero and E. Santiago-Delpin (1991) "Factors in a Meager Organ Donation Pattern of a Hispanic Population". *Transplantation Proceedings*, Vol. 23 (No. 2), pp.1799-1801.

Festinger, L. (1957) *A Theory of Cognitive Dissonance*. Stanford: Stanford University Press.

Festinger, L. and J. M.Carlsmith (1959) "Cognitive Consequences of Forced Compliance". *Journal of Abnormal and Social Psychology*, Vol. 58: 203-210.

Festinger, L., H. Riecken and S. Schachter (1956) *When Prophesy Fails*. Minneapolis: University of Minnesota Press.

Foucault, M. (1972) *Power/knowledge*. New York: Pantheon Books.

Fox, R.C. (1989) *The Sociology of Medicine: A Participant Observer's View*. Englewood Cliffs, New Jersey: Prentice-Hall.

Fox, R.C. (1993) "An Ignoble Form of Cannibalism". *The Kennedy Institute of Ethics Journal*, Vol. 3: 231-239.

Fox, R.C. (1959) *Experiment Perilous: Physicians and Patients Facing the Unknown*. Glencoe, Illinois: Free Press.

Fox, R.C. (1984) "Medical Morality is not Bioethics: Medical Ethics in China and the United States". *Perspectives in Biology and Medicine*, Vol. 27: 336-360.

Fox, R.C. (1988) *Essays in Medical Sociology. Journeys into the Field*. New Brunswick (USA) and Oxford (UK): Transaction Books.

Fox, R.C. (1990) "The Evolution of the American Bioethics" in Weisz, G. (ed.) *Social Science Perspective on Medical Ethics*. Dordrecht: Kluwer Academic Publishers.

Fox, R.C. (1994) "The Entry of U.S. Bioethics into the 1990s: A Sociological Analysis" in DuBose et al.

Fox, R.C. and J. Sweazey (1974) *The Courage to Fail. A social view of organ transplants and dialysis*. University of Chicago Press.

Fox, R.C. and J. Sweazey (with the assistance of J.C. Watkins) (1989) *Spare Parts*. New York: Oxford University Press.

Francis, D., R. Walker, R. Millar and G. Becker (1992) "Living related and living unrelated kidney transplantation using low-dose triple immunosuppression". *Transplantation Proceedings*, Vol. 24 (No.5), pp.1887-1888.

Freedman, J. (1965) "Long-term Behavioral Effects of Cognitive Dissonance". *Journal of Experimental Social Psychology*, Vol. 1:145-155.

Fulton, J., R. Fulton and R. Simmons (1977) "The Cadaver Donor and the Gift of Life" in R. Simmons, S. Klein and R. Simmons, *The Gift of Life*.

GALLUP (1993) "The American Public's Attitudes Toward Organ Donation and Transplantation. A Survey". *The Gallup Organization for The Partnership for Organ Donation*, Boston, Massachusetts.

Gennep van, A. (1977) *The Rites of Passage*. London: Routledge and Kegan Paul.

Gentleman, D., J. Easton and B. Jennet (1990) "Brain death and organ donation in a neurosurgical unit: audit of recent practice". *British Journal of Medicine*, Vol. 301 (24 November), 1203-1206.

Giddens, A. (1984) *The Constitution of Society*. Cambridge: Polity Press.

Glaser, A. and P. Strauss (1965) *Awareness of Dying*. Aldine Publishing Company.

Goffman, E. (1951) *Asylums*. New York: Anchor Books.

Goffman, E. (1967) *Interaction Ritual: Essays on Face-to-Face Behavior*. Garden City, NewYork: Anchor.

Goffman, E. (1974) *Frame Analysis: An Essay on the Organization of Experience*. Cambridge: Harvard University Press.

Gomez, P. and C. Santiago (1995) "La negativa familiar. Causas y estrategias". *Revista Española de Transplantacion* 3 (3): 334-335.

Groth, C.G. (1989) "Njurtransplantation i Sverige 25 år". *Läkartidning*, Vol. 86 (No. 52), pp. 4589-91.

Gubernatis, G. (1997) "Solidarity Model as Nonmonetary Incentive Could Increase Organ Donation and Justice in Organ Allocation at the Same Time". *Transplantation Proceedings*. Vol. 29, 3264-3266.

Gäbel et al. (1990) "The procurement of kidney for transplantation in Scandinavia". *Transplantation Proceedings*. Vol. 22: No. 2.

Gäbel, H. and B. Edström (1991) "Organ från avlidna för transplantation. Efterfrågan ökar men inte antalet donatorer". *Läkartidningen*, Vol. 90 (No. 4), 248-257.

Gäbel, H. and K. Lindskoug (1989) "Svensk enkät om organdonation och transplatation: Tva tredjedelar redo att ge organ: Besked till de anhöriga fran en tredjedel". *Läkartidningen*. Vol. 86:3681-3692.

Gäbel, H. and K. Lindskoug (1987b) "Malmö enkät om attityder till organdonation och transplantation: 65% kan tänka sig att donera organ men bara 2% har gett skriftlig besked". *Läkartidningen*, Vol. 84, pp.1065-1069.

Gäbel, H. and K. Lindskoug (1987a) "65% kan tänka sig att donera organs men bara 2% har gett skriftligt besked". *Läkartidningen*. Vol.84, pp.1065-1069.

Gäbel, H., B. Book, M. Larsson and G. Åstrand (1989) "The attitudes of young men to cadaveric donation and transplantation. The influence of background factors and information". *Transplantation Proceedings*. Vol. 21 (No.1) (February), pp. 1413-1414.

Gäbel, H., J.Ahonen, J. Sodaland and L. Lamm (1992) "Organ Procurement in Scandinavian Countries". *Transplantation Proceedings*. Vol. 24, pp. 265-266.

Haas, J.E. and T. Drabek (1970) "Community disaster and social system stress:a sociological perspective" in J.E. McGrath (ed.) *Social and psychological factors in stress*. New York: Holt, Rhinehart and Winston Inc.

Handelman, D. (1995) *Models and Mirrors: Toward an Anthropology of Public Events*. Cambridge: Cambridge University Press.

Hansson, M. (1992) *How Ethical is it to Let People Die on the Waiting Lists?* Project report. Department of Sociology, Uppsala University.

Heclo, H. (1987) *Policy and Politics in Sweden*. Philadelphia:Temple University Press.

Heider, F. (1958) *The Psychology of Interpersonal Relations*. New York: Wiley.

Heimer, C.A. (1992) "Doing Your Job and Helping Your Friends: Universalistic Norms about Obligations to Particular Others in Networks" in Nohria and Eccles.

Hellbom, K. (1988) *Hjärtslaget pa Karolinska Sjukhuset*. Stockholm.

Hewitt, M. (1991) "Bio-Politics and Social Policy: Foucault's Account of Welfare" in Featherstone et al. (eds).

Horton, R. and P. Horton (1991) "A model of willingness to become a potential organ donor". *Social Science and Medicine*. Vol. 33, No. 9, 1037-1051.

Hughes, T. P. (1983) *Networks of Power*. Baltimore: Johns Hopkins University Press.

Ibarra, H. (1992) "Structural Alignments, Individual Strategies and Managerial Action: Elements Toward a Network Theory of Getting Things Done" in Nohria and Eccles.

Inger, G. (1985) "Rätten över liv och över egen kropp", *Kungliga Humanistiska Vetenskaps-Samfundet i Uppsala. Årsbok 1985*, pp. 104-115. Annales Societatis Literarium Humaniorum Regiae Upsaliensis.

Ishibashi, M. (1992) "Present Status of Transplantations in Japan". *Transplantation Proceedings*. Vol. 24 (No. 5) (October), pp.1821-1823.

JAMA (1985) "The Organ Procurement Problem: Many causes, no easy solutions". (Medical News), Vol. 254 (No. 23), pp. 3285-3288.

Joerges, B. (1988) "Large Technical Systems: Concepts and Issues" in R. Mayntz and T. Hughes (eds) *The Development of Large Technical Systems*. Frankfurt: Campus Verlag.

Kanter, R.M. (1983) *The Change Masters*. New York: Simon & Schuster.

Kanter, R.M. (1988) "When a Thousand Flowers Bloom: Structural, Collective and Social Conditions for Innovation in Organizations" in B. M. Staw and L.L. Cummings (eds) *Research in Organizational Behavior*, Vol. 10. Greenwich, Connecticut: JAI Press.

Keatings, M. (1990) "The Biology of the Persistent Vegetative State: State, Legal, and Ethical Implications for Organ Transplantation:Viewpoints from Nursing". *Transplantation Proceedings*. Vol. 22 (No. 3), pp. 997-999.

Kuhn, W. (1990) "Psychiatric distress during stages of the heart transplant protocol". *The Journal of Heart Transplantation*. Vol. 9, pp. 25-9.

Lai, M.K., Huang, C. and S. Chu (1992) "Noncompliance in renal transplant recipients: Experience in Taiwan". *Clinical transplantation.*

Land, W. and J.B. Dossetor (eds) (1991) *Replacement Therapy: Ethics, Justice, Commerce*. First Joint Meeting of ESOT and EDTA/ERA. Munich. December. Springer Verlag.

Laurence, P. and J.W. Lorsch (1967) *Organization and environment: managing differentiation and integration*. Boston, Massachusetts.

Lee, P. and P. Kissner (1986) "Organ Donation and the Uniform Anatomical Gift Act". *Surgery*, November.

Locke, M. and C. Honde (1990) "Reaching consensus about death: Heart Transplants and Cultural Identity in Japan" in G. Weisz (ed.) *Social Science Perspectives on Medical Ethics*. Netherlands: Kluwer Academic Publishers.

Lynn, J. (1993) "Are the Patients Who Become Organ Donors Under the Pittsburgh Protocol for Non-Heart Beating-Donors Really Dead?". *The Kennedy Institute of Ethics Journal*. Vol. 3 (No. 2), pp.167-178.

Machado, Calixto (1992) "Reflections on the First International Symposium on Brain Death" (Havana, September 22-25, 1992).

Machado, N. (1990) "Risk and Risk Assessments in Organizations: The Case of An Organ Transplantation System". Paper Presented at the XII World Congress of Sociology, Session on Risk and Risk Management, Madrid, Spain, July, 1990.

Machado, N. (1992) "A Sociological Process Model of Organ Transplantation". *Human Systems Management*. Vol. 11, pp. 23-34.

Machado, N. (1995) "Incongruence and Tensions in Complex Organizations: The Case of An Organ Transplantation System". *Human System Management*. Vol.15, pp.55-71.

Machado, N. (1996a) *Using the Bodies of the Dead. Studies in Organization, Law and Social Process Related to Organ Transplantation*. Ph.D. Dissertation. Department of Sociology. Uppsala University.

Machado, N. (1996b) "The Swedish Transplant Acts: Sociological Considerations On Bodies and Giving". *Social Science and Medicine*. Vol. 42, No. 2:159-168.

Machado, N. and T.R. Burns (1998) "Complex Social Organization: multiple organizing modes, structural incongruence, and mechanisms of integration". *Public Administration* (Summer 1998), Vol. 76, No. 2.

Madsen, M., P. Asmundsson, I.B. Brekke, K. Höckerstedt, P. Kirkegaard, N.H. Persson and G. Tuvesson (1997) "Scandiatransplant: Organ Transplantation in the Nordic Countries 1996". *Transplantation Proceedings*. Vol. 29, pp. 3084-3090.

Malinowski, B. (1954) *Magic, Science, and Religion and Other Essays*. Garden City, New York: Doubleday.

March, J.G. and J.P. Olsen (1976) *Ambiguity and Choice in Organizations*. Oslo: Universitetsforlaget.

March, J.G. and J.P. Olsen (1984) "The New Institutionalism: Organizational Factors in Political Life". *American Political Science Review* 78:734-89.

Martyn, S. (1988) "Reconsidering request". *Hastings Center Report*. April/May.

Mauss, M. (1954) The Gift: Forms and Functions of Exchange in Archaic Societies. London: Cohen and West.

Mauss, M. (1979) *Sociology and Psychology*. London: Routledge and Kegan Paul.

Mayntz, R. (1989) "Reflections on Socio-technical Systems". Paper presented at FRN-SCASSS Conference on "*Technology and Society*", May, 1989, Uppsala, Sweden.

Mayntz, R. and T. Huges (eds) (1988) *The Development of Large Technical Systems*. Frankfurt: Campus Verlag.

McMaster, P. and A. Czerniak (1991) "Living Related Transplantation: A Note of Caution" in Land, W. and J.B. Dossetor (eds) *Organ Replacement Therapy: Ethics, Justice, Commerce*. First Joint Meeting of ESOT and EDTA/ERA. Munich. December. Springer Verlag.

Menzies, I. (1970) *The functioning of Social Systems as a Defence Against Anxiety*. London: The Tavistock Institute.

Michailakis, D. (1995) *Legislating Death. Socio-legal Studies of the Brain Death Controversy in Sweden.* Dissertation Uppsala University. Acta Universitatis Upsaliensis.

Michielsen, P. (1991) "Medical Risk and Benefit in Renal Donors: The Use of Living Donation Reconsidered" in Land, W. and J.B. Dossetor (eds) *Organ Replacement Therapy: Ethics, Justice, Commerce.* First Joint Meeting of ESOT and EDTA/ERA. Munich. December. Springer Verlag.

Miranda, A. and R. Matesanz (1996) "The potential organ donor pool. International figures" in Matesanz, R. and A. Miranda (eds) *Organ donation for transplantation: The Spanish Model.* ONT. Madrid: Grupo Aula Medica.

Moore, F. (1988) "Three ethical revelations: Ancient assumptions remodeled under pressure of transplantation". *Transplantation Proceedings*, 20 (Suppl. 1): 1061-1067.

Moore, J. (1988) "The gift of life: new laws, old dilemmas, and the future of organ procurement" in *Akron Law Review.* Spring: 443-487.

Nelson, E., J. Childress, J. Perryman, V. Robards, A. Rowan, M. Seely, S. Sterioff and M. Rovelli Swanson (1993) "Financial Incentives for Organ Donation A Report of the UNOS Ethics Committee Payment Subcommittee". UNOS, June 30, 1993.

Newsletter of *The Partnership for Organ Donation* (1994) "A Critical Look at Presumed vs. Informed Consent" in the Summer 1994 issue of "Progress Notes".

Nohria, N. and R. G. Eccles (eds) (1992) *Networks and Organizations: Structure, Form, and Action.* Boston: Harvard Business School Press.

NTAF. National Transplant Assistance Fund (1998) NTAF Information page, "http://www.transplantfund.org/homepage2.html".

O'Neill, R. (1996) "Organ Donation and Transplantation: An Overview of Current Ideas and Emergent Practices". Department of Sociology, University of Western Sydney, Macarthur, Australia.

Ouchi, W. (1980). "Markets, Bureaucaracies, and Clans". *Administration Science Quarterly*, Vol. 25, pp. 129-41.

Ouchi, W. (1991) "Markets, Bureaucracies and Clans" in Thompson, G., J. Frances, M. Levacic and J. Mitchell (eds).

Parsons, T. (1961) *Theories of society.* New York: Free Press.

Parsons, T. (1964) "Introduction" in Parsons (ed. and translator) *Max Weber: Social and Economic Organization.* New York: Free Press.

Peele, A.S. (1989) "The Nurse Role in Promoting the Rights of Donor's Families". *Nursing Clinics of North America.* Vol. 24, 4, December

1989:939.

Pelletier, M. (1992) "The organ donor family members' perception of stressful situations during the organ donation experience". *Journal of Advanced Nursing.* Vol. 17 (No. 1): 90-97.

Perrow, C. (1979) *Complex Organizations.* Glenview, Illinois: Scott, Foresman and Company.

Persijn, G. and A. van Netten (1997) "Public Education and Organ Donation". *Transplantation Proceedings.* Vol. 29, 1614-1617.

Pollock, F. and F. W. Maitland (1923) *The History of the English Law Before the Time of Edward I.* Cambridge: Cambridge University Press.

Powell, W.W. (1990) "Neither Market nor Hierarchy: Network Forms of Organization" in B. Staw (ed) *Research in Organizational Behavior,* Vol. 12. Greenwich, Connecticut: JAI Press, pp. 295-336.

Powell, W.W. and P. J. DiMaggio (eds) (1991) *The New Institutionalism in Organizational Analysis.* Chicago: University of Chicago Press.

Punch, J. (1997) "A More Technical Explanation of ABO Organ Matching" in Trans Web "http://www.transweb.org/faq/faq_abo_match".

Rettig, R. (1989) "The Politics of Organ Transplantation: A Parable of our Time". *Journal of Health Politics, Policy and Law.* Vol. 14, 1.

Roels, L., M. Roelants, T. Timmermans, K. Hoppenbrowers, E. Pillen and J. Bande-Knops (1997) "A Survey on Attitudes to Organ Donation Among Three Generations in a Country With 10 Years of Presumed Consent Legislation". *Transplantation Proceedings.* Vol. 29, 3224-3225.

Rynning, E. (1994) *Samtycke till medicinsk vård och behandling: en rättsvetenskaplig studie.* Uppsala: Iustus Forlag.

Sanner, M. (1989) see SOU 1984:81.

Sanner, M. (1991) *Den Döda Kroppen. Psykologiska Och Socialmedicinska Aspekter På Organdonation, Och Transplantation.* Dissertation. Department of Social Medicine. Uppsala Universitet.

Sanner, M. (1994) "Attitudes Toward Organ Donation and Transplantation. A Model for Understanding Reactions to Medical Procedures after Death". *Social Science and Medicine.* Vol. 38:1141-1152.

Santiago, C. and P. Gomez (1997) "Asking for the Family Consent". *Transplantation Proceedings.* Vol. 29: 1629-1630.

Scandiatransplant (1996) Verksamhetsberättelse för föreningen Scandiatransplant verksamhetsåret 1995/1996.

Schluchter, W. (1981) *The rise of Western Rationalism: Max Weber's*

Developmental History. Berkeley: University of California Press.

Schutt, G. and P. Schroeder (1993) "Population Attitudes Toward Organ Donation in Germany". *Transplantation Proceedings*. Vol. 25, No. 6 (December) 3127-3128.

Scott, R. W. (1981) *Organization: Rational, Natural, and Open Systems*. Englewood Cliffs, New Jersey:Prentice-Hall.

Self, D. and M. Olivarez (1993) "The influences of gender in conflicts of interest in the allocation of limited crucial care". *Journal of Critical Care*. March. 8 (1) 64-67.

Sells, A. (1991) "Voluntary Consent in Both Related and Unrelated Living Organ Donors" in Land, W. and J.B. Dossetor (eds) *Organ Replacement Therapy: Ethics, Justice, Commerce*. First Joint Meeting of ESOT and EDTA/ERA. Munich. December. Springer Verlag.

Simforoosh, N. et al. (1991) "Social Aspects of Kidney Donation in 300 Living Related and Unrelated Transplantations" in Land, W. and J.B. Dossetor.

Simmons, R., G.S.D. Klein and R.I. Simmons (1977) *Gift of Life: The Effect of Organ Transplantation on Individual, Family, and Societal Dynamics*. New York: John Wiley & Sons.

Sjölenius, B. (1989) *Hälso Och Sjukvårds Rätt*. Del I and II. Lund: Studentlitteratur.

Slapak, M. (1987) "Is There a Role for Kidney Transplantation in Developing Countries?". *Transplantation Proceedings*. Vol. 19 (No. 2) Suppl.2 (April) pp. 17-20.

Smith, A. and S. Kleinman (1989) "Emotions in medical School". *Social Psychology Quarterly*. Vol. 52 (No. 1): 56-69.

Sophie, L.R. (1983) *Heart Lung*, 12:261.

Steuer, J. and Bell, R. (1989) "Opting-in versus opting-out: an organ procurement dilemma". *Critical Care Nurse*. Vol. 9 (No.8).

Stinchcombe, A. (1985) "Contracts as hierarchical documents" in A. Stinchcombe and C. Heimer (eds) *Organizational Theory and Project Management*. Oslo: Norwegian University Press.

Surman, O. (1989) "Psychiatric Aspects of Organ Transplantation". *American Journal of Psychiatry* 146:8, August.

Sutherland, D. et al. (1991) "Medical Risks and Benefit of Pancreas Transplants from Living Related Donors" in Land, W. and J.B. Dossetor (eds) *Organ Replacement Therapy: Ethics, Justice, Commerce*. First Joint Meeting of ESOT and EDTA/ERA. Munich. December. Springer Verlag.

Sutton, C. (1998) *Studies in the Swedish alcohol discourse: definitions of social problems*. Ph.D. Dissertation. Department of Sociology. Uppsala University, Uppsala, Sweden.

Sweeting, H. and M. Gilhooly (1991) "Doctor, Am I Dead? A Review of Social Death in Modern Societies". *OMEGA.* Vol. 24(4) 251-269, 1991-92.

Taylor, C. (1989) *Sources of the Self: The Making of the Modern Identity.* Cambridge: Cambridge University Press.

Thibodeau, M. and Aronson, E. (1992) "Taking a Closer Look: Reasserting the Role of the Self-Concept in Dissonance Theory". *Personality and Social Psychology Bulletin.* Vol.18 (No. 5):591-602.

Thomas, L.V. (1975) *Antropologie de la mort.* Paris: Payot.

Thompson, G., J. Frances, R. Levacic and J. Mitchell (1991) *Markets, hierarchies, and networks: the coordination of social life.* London: Sage Publications.

Titmuss, R. (1970) *The Gift Relationship: From Human Blood to Social Policy.* Penguin Books.

Tomlinson, T. (1990) "Misunderstanding Death in A Respirator". *Bioethics.* Vol. 4, 253-264.

Toulmin, S. (1994) "Casuistry and Clinical Ethics" in E.R. DuBose, R.P.Hamel and L.J. O'Connell (eds).

Transplant 1991/1992. *Official report on Transplantation Activities of the Council of Europe.* Edited by the Foundation Marcel Mérieux, Lyon, France.

Trist, E. (1981) *The Evolution of Socio-technical Systems: a conceptual framework and action research program.* Toronto: Ontario Ministry of Labour.

Turner, B. S. (1984) *The Body and Society. Explorations in Social Theory.* London: Basil Blackwell.

Turner, B.S. (1991) "Recent Developments in the Theory of the Body" in Featherstone et al. (eds).

Turner, B.S. (1992) *Regulating Bodies: Essays in Medical Sociology.* London: Routledge.

Turner, V. (1969) *The Ritual Process: Structure and Anti-Structure.* Ithaca, New York: Cornell University Press.

Tännsjö, T. (9/4/90) *"Värför kräva samtycke?"*. Dagens Nyheter Debatt.

UNOS Annual Report (1996) *The U.S. Scientific Registry of Transplant Recipients and The Organ Procurement and Transplantation Network*

Transplant Data 1988-1995. United Network for Organ Sharing.

Veatch, R. (1993a) "The Impending Collapse of the Whole Brain Definition of Death". *Hastings Center Report*, pp. 18-24.

Veatch, R. (1993b) "Forgoing Life-Sustaining Treatment: Limits To Consensus". *The Kennedy Institute of Ethics Journal.* Vol. 3 (No.1): 1-19.

Vicusi, W., W. Magat and A. Forrest (1988) "Altruistic and Private Valuations in Risk Reduction". *Journal of Policy Analysis & Management*, p. 227.

Waitzkin, H. (1989) "A Critical Theory of Medical Discourse: Ideology, Social Control, and the Processing of Social Context in Medical Encounters". *Journal of Health and Social Behavior.* Vol. 30: 220-239.

Waitzkin, H., T. Britt and C. Williams (1994) "Narratives of Aging and Social Problems in Medical Encounters with Older Persons". *Journal of Health and Social Behavior.* Vol. 35: 322-348.

Walzer, M. (1983) *Spheres of Justice: a Defence of Pluralism and Equality.* Basic Books, New York.

Weber, M. (1968) *Economy and society.* New York: Bedminister.

Weber, M. (1977) *From Max Weber: Essays in Sociology.* Edited with an introduction by H.H. Gerth and C.W. Mills. Routledge and Kegan Paul. Oxford.

Weick, K.E. (1979) *The Social Psychology of Organizing.* New York: Random House.

Wellman, B. and S. D. Berkowitz (eds) (1988) *Social Structures: A Network Approach.* New York: Cambridge University Press.

Wicklund, R. and J. Brehm (1976) *Perspectives on Cognitive Dissonance.* Hillsdale, N.J.: Lawrence Erlbaum Associates.

Wiley, N. (1994) *The Semiotic Self.* Cambridge: Polity Press.

Winner, L. (1977) *Autonomous Technology.* Cambridge, Massachusetts. MIT Press.

Withington, P., M. Siegler and C. Broelsch (1991) "Living Donor Nonrenal Organ Transplantation: A Focus on Living Renal Orthoptic Liver Transplantation" in Land, W. and J.B. Dossetor (eds) *Organ Replacement Therapy: Ethics, Justice, Commerce.* First Joint Meeting of ESOT and EDTA/ERA. Munich. December. Springer Verlag.

Wolf, Z.R. (1988) "Nursing Rituals". *Canadian Journal of Nursing Research.* Vol. 20: 59-69.

Wolf, Z.R. (1988) *Nurses At Work: the Sacred and the Profane.* Philadephia:

University of Philadelphia.

Wolf, Z.R. (1990) "Nurses Experiences Giving Post-Mortem Care to Patients Who Have Donated Organs: A Phenomenological Study". *Transplantation Proceedings.* Vol. 22 (No.3): 1019-1020.

Wolfe, A. (1989) *Whose keeper?   Social Science and Moral Obligation.* University of California Press.

Yanaga, et al. (1989) "Personal experience with the procurement of 132 liver allografts". *Transplant.* Vol. 2:137-142.

Youngner, S. (1990) "Organ Retrieval: Can We Ignore the Dark Side?". *Transplantation Proceedings.* Vol. 22 (No. 3) (June) pp. 1014-1015.

Youngner, S. (1992a) "Defining Death: A Superficial and Fragile Consensus". *Archives of Neurology.* Vol. 49:570-572.

Youngner, S. (1992b) "Organ Donation and Procurement" in J. Craven and G. Rodin (eds) *Psychiatric Aspects of Organ Donation.* Oxford: Oxford University Press.

Youngner, S. (1992c) "Psychological Impediments to Procurement". *Transplantation Proceedings.* Vol. 24 (No. 5) (Oct): 2159-2161.

Youngner, S., C. Landefelt, C. Colton, B. W. Jukinialis and M. Leary (1989) "Brain Death and Organ Retrieval: A Cross-Sectional Survey of Knowledge and Concepts Among Health Professionals". *JAMA.* Vol. 261 (No. 15): 2205-2210.

Zajonc, R. (1968a) "Cognitive Theories in Social Psychology" in G. Lindzey and E. Aronson (eds) *The Handbook of Social Psychology.* Reading, Massachusetts: Addison-Wesley.

Zajonc, R. (1968b) "Cognitive Organization and Processes" in D.L. Sills (ed.) *Encyclopedia of The Social Sciences,* Vol. 5, pp. 615-622. New York: Macmillan and Company and Free Press.

Zerubavel, E. (1993) *The Fine Line.* Chicago:University of Chicago.

Zussman, R. (1992) *Intensive Care: Medical Ethics and the Medical Profession.* Chicago, London: The University of Chicago Press.

Öström, M. and Eriksson, A. (1989) *Traffic Fatalities Among Women in Northern Sweden* in M. Valverius (ed.) *Women, Alcohol, Drugs and Traffic.* Proceedings of the International Workshop. September 29-30, 1989.

Index

Printed and bound by CPI Group (UK) Ltd, Croydon, CR0 4YY

21/10/2024

01777084-0002